Our Presence Has Roots

The Ongoing Story of Deohaeko Support Network

Janet Klees

Resources Supporting Family and Community Legacies Inc.

Toronto, Ontario 2005

Library and Archives Canada Cataloguing in Publication
Klees, Janet, 1959-

Our presence has roots: the ongoing story of Deohaeko Support Network/Janet Klees.

Includes bibliographical references and index.
ISBN 1-55307-017-8

1. Deohaeko Support Network. 2. Rougemount Co-operative Homes. 3. Developmentally disabled--Services for--Ontario--Durham (Regional municipality). 4. Developmentally disabled--Housing--Ontario--Durham (Regional municipality). I. Resources Supporting Family and Community Legacies Inc. II. Title.

HV1570.5.C32O58 2005   362.196'8588'00971356   C2005-902691-X

To contact the author, write or call:

Janet Klees
c/o the Publisher
Resources Supporting Family and Community Legacies Inc.
11 Miniot Circle
Toronto, ON M1K 2K1 Canada
(416) 264 4665; Deohaeko (905) 509-5654
janet@legacies.ca
www.legacies.ca

The families of **Deohaeko Support Network** would like to thank the **Ontario Trillium Foundation** for their financial contribution to this book.

Printed in Canada by Webcom Limited.

Dedication

Dedicated to

those who have entrusted me with their stories—

Jonathan, Tiffany, Caroline Ann, Brenda, John, Donna and Rob.

Thank you.

And to the three

whose stories encircle my life, ground me

and keep me well—

Bram, Joanna and Harry.

Thank you.

I love you.

Table of Contents

Acknowledgements

This is a book about place, and its writing helped me to discover much about place in my own community. I want to thank those who allowed me to use space away from home for writing and reflection. In this sense, the book carries an essence of these community places where I found welcome and necessary solitude, elements that are increasingly hard to find in our rushed and connected world. Ironically, just as I was looking for 'places apart' from which I could do my writing, I discovered places connected to my community, where the welcome and understanding of the hosts provided the temporary sense of 'apart' that I needed. I thank *Dayspring*, the l'Arche Daybreak retreat house in Richmond Hill, where I accomplished many of my larger blocks of writing, cushioned and inspired by the solitude of a space set apart from the rush of the urban world around. I thank Father William Cruse and the members of the Church of Epiphany just behind our home. They allowed me to use their little room three or four times a week across two periods of writing time—close enough to home to be a part of home life, but far enough away for the isolation I need to write. I thank Johan and Olga, around the corner from our house, who allowed me to write in their home several times a week during the course of one summer while they crossed Canada in their trailer home. I thank Deb Thivierge for a wonderful editing weekend at her new cottage home north of Orillia, where she fed me treats and created space and time for me to work for hours on end.

I thank the families of Deohaeko Support Network for the continued privilege of being witness to their lives and their stories. The parents have spent so many hours with me and have shared so much in ways that have shaped and changed my own view of the world forever. They are ever the hidden editors behind my words and the final judges of how I tell their stories. They are kind, insightful, and unrelenting in their quest for a good life for their sons and daughters. This book is the better because of the example they set before me. The seven young men and women who are the heart of this book, just as the last, let me know in many ways that they recognize and welcome the depth of my caring and my respect for them. In a world where most of us can never be sure that others know how much we care, I *know*, and this is a profound gift.

I thank my dedicated group of editors. The families of Deohaeko approved the first draft, especially Linda Dawe, who gave me wise comments on several tricky sections, Harriet Salmers who gave me detailed proofing of the whole document, and Helen Dionne who gave me support and thought for the whole book. Diane Huson, my friend since Grade 3, who accompanies me in my work in many ways, gave enthusiastic support and tireless thinking from beneath her many hats: Supporter, friend, and circle member. Jack Yates, who has an exceptional ear and eye for the right word in the right place is largely responsible for a smoother, more succinct document than might otherwise have been. In addition, his gentle, accurate challenges from his strong value base have ensured for a stronger, more coherent voice. Peter Dill helped with the pattern and overall shape of the book, in his unfailing guidance to write an ending which includes the struggle and the fears, rather than a perfect ending. And Harry van Bommel, my best friend, husband, and fellow writer who edited every version, ever the champion of my work and this group of people, never allowing that the challenges that we face overshadow the strength of our accomplishments.

There is another group of people who deserve to publicly know of my appreciation for their time and presence in my life during the writing of this book. These are the many individuals with whom I have had conversations about the various topics touched upon in this book. Each conversation has led me to re-evaluate ideas, gain insights, struggle to articulate my deepest feelings, and seek a deeper understanding of the work that has called me forth. These people can be found among the Supporters of Deohaeko families, among the members of the Values Group in Pickering, and among the many people engaged in the work of building community in Durham Region, Scarborough and wider abroad. If you have ever been in conversation with me on these matters, then you may recognize yourselves as a part of this book. Thank you.

Finally, I want to say thank you to my family—Joanna, Bram and Harry—who have been with me in every point along the way writing this book. They have missed me and managed without me during my writing retreats, writing weekends, and editing binges. They have discussed many aspects of life and work at Rougemount and understand well the intricacies of this book. More importantly, as we live and grow together as a family, I cannot help but bring some of the ideas and beliefs that have been shaped by Deohaeko back to my family. In the end, Bram and Joanna are my greatest tangible proof that community *is* better when everyone is welcomed, recognized and included. This, they accept as self-evident and are heart-warmingly incredulous when they learn that not everyone thinks the same way they do. Thank you for the time you have given me to write, your interest in what I do, and all of the times in between when I get to be nothing more—and nothing less—than a mom to my favourite kids in the world!

And thank you to my mainstay, my greatest supporter, and the guy who centres my life today and for the past 20 years—Harry, you're the best!

At the Heart of Deohaeko

Deohaeko refers to the name given to the Spirit Supporters of Life. It pays homage to aboriginal people who occupied this area since before the coming of the Europeans.

At the heart of Deohaeko, is the belief that people who have never been able to dream of having homes of their own, will come to live in those homes among other people who will welcome them. In discovering and nurturing everyone's gifts, a strong community will evolve, so that the dignity, uniqueness, freedom and participation of each individual will be honoured and facilitated in a natural, neighbourly fashion, and that the community will be seen as a preferred place to live.

Like all members of our community, each of the individuals supported through Deohaeko has unique gifts to be offered. Deohaeko is committed to inviting, encouraging, welcoming and sustaining a level of community inclusion, participation and friendship that will make caring for one another a natural part of life in both the co-operative and greater community.

Firstly, Deohaeko will assist members of Rougemount Co-operative to foster a spirit of mutual neighbourhood support—the principle upon which this co-operative is established. All community members will find ways to welcome the gifts and talents of their neighbours.

Secondly, on an individual basis, each participant will be supported by family, friends, new neighbours, and personal supporters, if needed, to establish a home and share in both the co-operative community and the larger Durham Region community. Deohaeko sees the creation of a support network for each individual as a way to make possible the welcoming, the initial relationship building, the discovery of gifts and the nurturing of community.

Deohaeko will respond, respect, endure, and commit to the evolving community. It will be a communicator for the individuals it supports within the community.

Deohaeko joins with Rougemount in reaching for our dream of intentional community—a community where all members are welcomed, where all people share their gifts and find ways to support one another, and where lasting personal friendships grow.

From our Deohaeko archives

Introduction

This book is part of an ongoing story about community, about change, and about a group of families in Pickering, Ontario who are determined to make their community a changed and better place for all. It is the story of the giving of a gift of relationship and community that is not possible for the whole community to see or understand immediately, but one that these families know will strengthen and enrich the entire community as they choose to receive and partake of it.

This book is about the various ways the families of Deohaeko Support Network think about, plan for and make sure that the presence and gifts of their family members with disabilities are able to endure, well rooted in a nurturing environment in their community. This book is a record of our achievements so far, a reflection of what we have learned through both achievements and failures, and a guide to how and what we are trying to do now.

I continue to hold a unique position within this story. For the past ten years, I have had the privilege and the pleasure of walking with each of these families in my role as paid coordinator for the family group. At the same time, part of my life is also absorbed in my own family journey that is complementary, but different. These two experiences have given me some unique opportunities. I have come to know some of the day-to-day experiences of the families, to be closer than most others to the group, and, in fact, a part of the group at many times. My role with individual families allows me to become very intimate with different parts of their story as it unfolds. At the same time, because I accompany them but am not one of the families, I am also able to step back and reflect on the whole picture from time to time. My role with the whole of the family group often means that I step back and hold the whole picture, so that the families can make sound decisions about next steps. This book reflects this same dichotomy of experience, as both insider and outsider to the group.

The voice in this story is a shared voice with the families when I describe our common experiences. However, the analysis that arises in parts of this story is my own—the result of the reflection, experiences, discussions, and shaping that I do when I step back a bit from my direct experience. In this way, this story is my own, although shaped by our common experience and many hours of joint reflection on our journey. Any one of the families could write their own understanding of the meaning of our experiences together, and it would be different from, but just as valid, as my own.

This book has been written for other families curious about our journey, and for families, allies and Supporters (Note: *I use the upper case letter to indicate a paid role, as differentiated from supporters generally who are supportive people in the person's life who may or may not be paid*) who are dedicated to being a part of their family member's journey. It can be read for the enjoyment and the understanding of the whole of the story. It can also be used to understand and learn some practical approaches and strategies that families and their supporters can apply to their own unique situations. We spend time talking to families across Ontario and from around the world. We always want to emphasize that our story is not essentially about our co-operative home, but about how we come to think about and help individuals live unique, meaningful, contributing lives within the hearts of their community, wherever they are and whatever their starting point. This book is not a recipe for success, but a guide and a pathway of our particular journey in progress. Others may follow many or none of our steps in their journey. For some this will be simply a good story. For others, it may be an inspiration or a catalyst for new action. And for others again, it might provide some of the practical ideas that have been missing.

Deohaeko Support Network is a family group in Durham Region, Ontario, which is comprised of eight families. Each family has an adult son or daughter with a developmental disability, and this person is the catalyst for family and supportive allies to be thinking and acting on ways to build strong community in Durham. The families of Deohaeko (rhymes with 'a long time ago') function as a group to think about the support and the lives of their family member, but they act individually to implement and help their family member lead a unique and meaningful life.

Our book about Deohaeko's first seven years, *We Come Bearing Gifts*, described the building of our foundations. It was about the actual designing of a housing co-operative and an intentional community that many people, including the sons and daughters of the founding families, could call home. But even more, it was fundamentally about building support that would work in order for people to live good lives. It was about our thinking and actions around relationships, circles, support, community roles and connections, and the future. That future is now. Many people see the vibrant, busy lives of the individuals who receive support through Deohaeko Support Network and think that our work and goals have been achieved. We are proud of what we have accomplished, but in many ways feel that the tough work is still to be done.

Our work over the first seven years caused most members of society little effort or thought to accept to our presence and contributions. But now we want much more. We are just beginning to work at deep issues that our quick-paced, image-focused society hardly recognizes and does not want to face. We want to acknowledge and work with frailties and vulnerabilities that will not go away, poverty that will not recede into full-time jobs, support requirements that will not disappear with education or therapy, and futures that cannot be left to programs and agencies to manage. In many ways, by delving deeper, we are going against the tide. Rather than being content with a façade of achievement and success, for the sake of our children and of our communities, we want to work on rooting ourselves in real community. And then, we want the community to recognize that it needs the presence of its vulnerable members in order to be ready for the future.

And so, our work and our focus have changed. In the first seven years, our focus on *relationship* brought us to meeting people, ensuring welcome and becoming friendly. Now we're talking about truly seeing people in all their fullness, making real effort, personal relationships and commitment.

Before, with *circles*, we did the inviting, gathering and planning. Now we're working on it again, filling in gaps, trouble shooting, and aiming for formats and members that work for people individually into the future. We are slowly finding ways to talk to each other about uncertain futures and trying to find ways to ask circle members to join in answering the parents' question, "what happens when I die?" We are grappling with futures where parents are not the key organizers and coordinators.

For the first seven years, in *community roles and connections*, we worked on presence and real participation. Now we are talking about and working toward establishing identity, receiving recognition and belonging. We know that families and supporters need to understand and work well with the concepts of place, presence, role and relationships with other people. We are looking to connections that will root the person within their community by relationship, place and genuine contribution.

Our previous work on *support* focused our efforts on creative interviewing, good orientation, and recognizing natural supports. Now we need to work at developing new kinds of paid relationships, recruiting in a very different world, encouraging and challenging natural supports, and imagining how it will all hold together without the parents.

Our work has brought us to that *future* that we knew would come. Two family board members have now died, and all other family members are feeling the energy drain and health constraints placed on them by another ten years of life and work. In the beginning, we imagined and built a good place to live and we painstakingly secured funding to keep us there. In 2002 we established an endowment fund to address our long-term financial requirements for direct support, and now we need to focus on filling it up while our stamina remains. We have outlined (many in writing) clear visions of a good life for each of our sons and daughters, and now we need to re-write them in detail, making sure that they are understood by those taking on significant roles in the future. This too, is work that goes against the tide. In our society, most people do not prepare in significant ways for their death, except financially, and spend little time talking this through with others. We are beginning to see that we must push through this wall of inhibition and have many and deep conversations with others to secure a good future for our family member.

So, in many aspects, these are the tough years, focusing on building from the roots up for a strong and healthy future. This is our story about what we think about, how we keep focus, and what this next stage is all about for us. What keeps us going through this difficult work during our latter years? Three things in particular keep us focused on our work.

One reason that our energy and focus continues the work that we have set out, is that we believe that our family members with a disability bring gifts and qualities which are precisely those that our communities need in order to ensure their health and strength into the future. Our fast-moving society needs good reasons to slow down, to reflect on experiences and impacts, to take time to build ways that include rather than exclude. Our communities need all of their members. It's in figuring out how to welcome and include people. That the gifts of vulnerable members are uncovered and the gifts of typical community members come to light.

The **second reason** that we work so hard to ensure that our sons and daughters are well established as valued citizens within their community is that we are aware of how terribly vulnerable they truly are. In general, we know that our family members are not automatically accorded high status, value or even well cared for in our society. If people think of them at all, it is to assume that they are cared for by some agency or system with the responsibility for doing so. Still others take advantage of them, assume that they require a lesser standard of living than most people, or view them as a way to make a living for themselves through a pay cheque from a social service or government agency. As long as our family members and others like them remain so vulnerable in our communities, we and others who come to care, must advocate fiercely on their behalf so that the gifts, now unseen by so many, may be offered and received by society.

Since this way of welcoming, recognizing and including is so obviously not the typical way we see in our community, it is evident that our communities need some good models and pathways to contemplate or follow. This constitutes the **third reason** as to why we are putting time and effort into this way of living. We strive to be a living model of the possibilities that exist when a community learns how to include and embrace some of its most vulnerable members. We have successes that we all feel good about and we have failures and challenges from which we all learn. Much is far from perfect, and yet we endure. Our community is stronger because of the example of a small group of people who strive to build a better way every hour, every day.

We have learned some important lessons over the past 15 years. Some of them are lessons first learned in our early years. Others have been learned more recently.

We have learned that families who value the concept of relationship and community roles highly, put their efforts and time in those directions, take on the difficult asking role, and are rewarded with solid achievements. Neighbours, citizens and co-workers come forward in friendship and various forms of freely-given relationship. Individuals are less well rooted where the family's other values place competing obligations on time and energy.

We have learned that it is harder and harder to find places conducive to belonging where people can belong. There is a whole new 'franchise-strip heaven' of stores, businesses and fast food franchises just east of the Rougemount Co-operative. There is little chance for flexibility, little tolerance of difference, and little valuing of slowing down the pace of life in those places. There is little opportunity for employees who feel willing or able to change their routine and permit a relationship to grow. Employees are dressed uniformly, have prescribed job duties, and are timed to the *nth* degree to ensure that they do not drift into time-wasting, profit-threatening individuality and relationship.

We have learned that you have to become able to see the cracks in the facade and act on them. In actual fact, not everyone buys into the productive, consumerism society. We're looking for environmental groups, neighbourhood groups, social committees, and local event teams—all eager for volunteers, companions and fellow enthusiasts. And even within the franchises themselves, we work hard to discover individuals who still want to make a difference and make it possible for someone to have a job accommodated to their strengths and abilities.

We have learned that the world is in constant flux and change while we all crave stability. A circle of support with relatively more neighbours and family members, and a few paid Supporters who come and go, can be a wonderful place for all its members to savour regular times of stability and familiarity.

We have learned that opportunities continually begin and end. It can be an exhausting process if you think that there is an end in sight and that each situation will remain perfect forever. It is more helpful to believe that there is no end, only more opportunities...thank goodness.

We have learned that vigilance is ever necessary. If things are not moving forward, they are likely moving backwards. Signs of healthy relationships and environments include lots of enthusiasm, people brimming with new ideas, and people bursting to tell stories. Signs of trouble include periods of silence (during which you are vainly hoping that all is well), small problems that seem bigger to others than they do to you, lack of ideas, and no stories to tell at the end of the day.

We have learned that we need to be conscious of the need to safeguard what we have and what we value. It can all be lost and lost quickly, with a sudden illness, a change in living situations or a change in funding.

We have learned to speak to others often and freely. We share our story. In doing so, each time we are strengthened. Somehow, we are refreshed when we repeat stories of past success. We are forgiving of ourselves and others as we reveal past difficulties. New ideas and ways of seeing things arise as we articulate life and joys and worries.

And perhaps, in the end, this is what this book is all about. It's another chance for us to tell our stories. In telling our stories, we can move from current struggles to past achievements, even if for only a short time. But it's important not to forget to celebrate just because our current struggles seem more urgent to us right now. The problems immediately in front of us will always seem more urgent, but they are not necessarily more important. Scott Ritchie, a young man from Scotland, once said that it is a mistake to let the urgent drive out the important. Past successes and reminding ourselves of how to do things right are important and worthy of celebration.

Growing things are important to me and a gardening analogy may be clarifying. I love flowers and weeds and natural spaces of any kind with a passion. I don't know enough about the basics to really be effective in a formal garden, but I find ways to naturalize the spaces around me. I have a casual, unstructured approach to gardening. I think that I've had this approach to formal gardening because I've not felt that gardens or flowers need me in particular to survive. However, the natural and wild spaces around our little creek, the Taylor-Massey, seemed threatened by garbage and neglect when we first moved into our neighbourhood years ago. Our family's response was to quickly organize an annual neighbourhood creek clean up that continues to this day. When the trees along the creek seemed threatened by eroding floodwaters, we started an annual tree planting. Perhaps it was recognizing what we loved and cherished was at risk, that built within me an energy to action.

And when I think about it, when I heard the stories of Tiffany, Brenda, Donna, Jon, Caroline Ann, Rob and John ten years ago, they touched my heart to action as well. I think my passion was ignited when I realized that their gifts, contributions and very presence were at risk for want of a secure place within their communities. But along with the others, in order to do a good job, I have had to learn the basics. I have had to figure out how things work and how they might be done differently. In many ways, this book is my primer to structuring my passion and making it more effective. The most important lesson I have learned is that you cannot be a good gardener unless you have a passion for it. You cannot be a good community builder unless that which you build is passionately important to you.

The communities that I seek to build, encourage and strengthen are not just for Brenda, Donna, Rob, Jon, Caroline Ann, Tiffany and members of the Pickering community in which they live. They are also for my children, Bram and Joanna, my Scarborough neighbours, and others who may learn and grow from our experiences. My Deohaeko experience teaches me deeply about the gifts communities risk losing by not including all of their members. My children and my own neighbourhood experiences teach me about what we have to gain when everyone is included.

The story of our family group is ongoing. Out of necessity, I needed to put an endpoint to this part of the story in order to get it finished. Most of the story told in this book ends with 2003. As it turns out, there is a certain logic to this decision and a distinct pattern emerges as I write the last chapter and look back over the last eight years and forward to the next. As this book goes to publication, I see that we are already well into the next phase of our journey—handing over the securing of good lives now and in the future for our sons and daughters to another generation. Once again, we are meeting new situations and challenges for which we do not have ready answers. Once again we will have to rely on what we know and what we believe in as we carefully forge new ways in circumstances that are very different from those we had foreseen.

Faith, I have come to believe, is a trustworthy bridge between a knowable past and an uncertain future. It is the act of going through the right motions for the right reasons and believing that you will find sufficient secure footholds amidst the current uncertainty to see you to the other side. Faith and hard work saw us through our initial years, allowed us to build and grow through these past years, and will certainly see us into the future.

Section 1
Cultivating the Soil

Chapter 1: An Update
Chapter 2: Philosophy at the Foundation

I remember growing up on Vancouver Island atop the sandy soil layers that are cradled between the ocean edges and the rocky island peaks. Back then, I thought that dirt was dirt, but now I recall my father bemoaning the sandy soil and wishing for a bit of the dark, rich loam of his native Holland. Not content to merely accept his lot, my father spent hours every year, collecting kitchen scraps, preparing compost and digging its nutrients into the sandy soil. It is clear to me that he thought that things would grow more or less abundantly depending with which kind of 'dirt' one was blessed. And when you don't have the right 'stuff', the right soil, you go ahead and make your own with the raw materials at hand.

When we cultivate the soil in preparation for gardening, we are in the act of refining and improving the soil so that it is of maximum benefit to the plants and garden at hand. This is, however, in itself a second step to gardening although it is the point that we often refer to as the beginning of the gardening process. The absolute beginning of gardening is the assumption that one has some soil and some plants or seeds, and some water with which to work. At the same time, these are the items that one almost always takes for granted.

The people involved with Deohaeko Support Network have, through their own hard work, blend of personality and timing, and tenacity, cultivated their own unique grade of soil. They are good, hard working people who are rooted themselves in community life in many ways. This, then, is where they also want their children to be. They have talked long and hard together, enough to know that they are all moving in the same direction. Their imagination and energy have enabled their sons and daughters to thrive in their homes and community.

The families of Deohaeko bring two nourishing ingredients to this soil. In the first place they bring their stories. They have a strong sense of story. They tell a good story about their own lives, and those of their sons and daughters. They also hold the beginning of new stories— stories of dreams and hopes and fears that they are willing to share with one another. They tell these stories and use them to nourish others as well. Other family, friends and support people begin to join in the telling and understanding of the stories. Their stories become our stories. As we articulate, we are able to reflect and plan some more, to move a little farther down the path. In this section, the chapter on updates of the families is only one version of how this is done. Many other stories will follow in the rest of the book.

The second ingredient that we have brought to nourish and enrich the soil is a carefully articulated set of principles that provide a clear guide on complex issues. These lend a structure and reliability to all the work that we do. Even when we make mistakes and leave the path, this strong set of principles is a way that we can pull each other and ourselves back in line.

Interestingly enough, these two ingredients of telling stories and articulating principles are interwoven as they developed in real time and also within this section of the book. Bringing readers up to date on the lives of the families of Deohaeko and of the group itself has led us to great questions of principle and direction, based on our values, beliefs and experiences. Grappling with and resolving these principles has always been a question of story for us. Every principle that we have set down to paper springs up out of countless stories that stem from our lives and those of our family members. We are a practical group and mostly have little time to wax philosophic about ideas that never hit the ground. Instead, we have worked out a set of principles that will guide us in the very territory where we often run into trouble. The second chapter in this section will show just how intertwined our principles and our stories really are. We think of many of our stories as principles in action.

Chapter 1
An Update

Who are we?
We are citizens shaping a better world.
We are parents,
led by our sons and daughters.
Our love makes us open to their gifts, and
vulnerable to their fragile presence.

Their fragility teaches us
to build circles,
value relationship,
find welcome in community spaces,
think of mutual support,
plan for the future, and
embrace life.

This we do in the name of love.

(1997-2004) Eight Years Later

The families of Deohaeko Support Network first came together in 1989, in response to a question posed by Peter Dill, who then was with the nearby Ajax-Pickering-Whitby Association for Community Living, of which most families were members. The question was simple: "Where will your children live in the future?" But it was obviously the right question because about 75 families came to that first discussion. Over time, the group sifted down to the twelve families who would make a commitment to each other to work together on a common answer to that question over the long term.

These families researched and discussed, far into many late nights, the various options they felt were possible, or probable or desirable. They realized that their discussions led them as much to discussions of *how* their sons and daughters would live in the future as *where*. They finally brought the where and the how together by designing and finding ways to build a 105-unit housing co-operative with an intentional community at the edge of Pickering's Rouge Valley.

These considerable efforts led to a building and a housing community that the families felt many people could and would call 'home'.

As described in our first book, *We Come Bearing Gifts (1996),* the families originally wore dual hats in their founding roles of both the Rougemount Co-operative and the Deohaeko Support Network. Over time, as planned, the families handed over their founding board roles in the Rougemount Co-operative to the members who lived in the co-operative community. They continued in their role as directors of Deohaeko Support Network and enjoyed the challenges of the unique role that Deohaeko held within the co-operative. Deohaeko's mission included several simultaneous roles. First of all, they were to be thoughtful and planful about the lives of their sons and daughters in both the co-operative and the greater community, to ensure that they were afforded the opportunities to live full, meaningful lives within the heart of their communities. Secondly, they were welcomed with two places at the Rougemount board in recognition of their wisdom and commitment gained over the designing and development of both the physical building and the intentional community spirit. This was a brand new option for co-operatives to follow, and Deohaeko and Rougemount members were proud to take advantage of this option. Thirdly, Deohaeko committed itself to being 'keepers of the flame'—the formal or informal watchdog of the spirit of community in the co-operative.

By the end of *We Come Bearing Gifts,* we had followed the Deohaeko families for the first seven years of their mutual journey. There were then eleven families and ten people receiving support and choosing to make

Rougemount Housing Co-operative their home. Rougemount was a thriving community of some 200 people who represented the full range of typical singles and families in Durham Region. The intentional community component of Rougemount provided challenges to its members, but neighbourliness and connections ran high. Individuals with disabilities were living in one, two or three bedroom units and were all engaged in a range of work, volunteer and civic roles during the week. They had a growing range of friendships and new relationships and were just beginning to dream in bigger ways for their future. Paid support, although not at optimal levels, came through annualized funding from the Ontario Ministry of Community and Social Services and was individualized by Deohaeko as it was funnelled through a local transfer payment agency (Durham Association for Family Respite). Families continued to share funds during times of need throughout the year. All support was one-to-one and so individualized for each person, and Deohaeko had started a policy of not recruiting paid support from among the members of the co-operative, as payment was seen as undermining the spirit of co-operation in the community.

Eight years later, where are we? In great part, that is the story of this book. But a basic overview of the families, the lives of individuals, and Deohaeko priorities will be helpful in order to help readers situate the stories into a larger framework.

The People

The lives of the individual people of Deohaeko who receive support will be detailed throughout the book.

Brenda Gray continues to live in her apartment with the patio facing the sidewalk, and fills her days in many ways. Four years ago, she successfully petitioned City Hall to be named as environmental steward of a small local park site. This important role gives shape and context to her week. At the best of times, she visits her site three or four times a week for a variety of environmental tasks. Brenda's new computer, complete with digital camera, should add new aspects to the opportunities of the site. She is also a regular at a local wildlife sanctuary, has taken up oil and watercolour painting, and enjoys lengthy chapter books read aloud. Brenda has developed a special place in her heart for young Matthew, Donna's son, and surprises him with toys and treats all the time. Hilda, Brenda's next door neighbour, continues to share tea with Brenda most days at 4:00, as she has for the past ten years. Over the past year, Brenda's brothers and sister and their families have taken on new roles around financial matters, Supporter invoicing, and coordination of support. Brenda loves the days when it's her sister-in-law, Barb's day to come in, write Supporter cheques, and spend some time with her. Brenda continues to challenge us to provide the most genuine and sensitive of paid Supporters, and to dream up of new ways to provide support that does not feel scheduled, intrusive or too obvious.

Caroline Ann Dionne celebrated her 40th birthday last year with a huge Karaoke party and over 75 well-wishers and friends. She went with three other women on a long-dreamed trip to England and Scotland. She is the first of the group to articulate a desire for 'home' to be defined in different terms than those afforded at Rougemount. Her circle is proud to have been able to listen to her deeply, and support her with her move into her own self-contained apartment within a house (her definition of home) in a neighbourhood where she is known and loved. She now lives in a separate apartment in the home of her parents. Caroline Ann has also realized other dreams over the years. She produced two CD vocal recordings. She has made two retreats to the Loretto Centre for connection and renewal, and plans for more in the future. She has made a thoughtful decision to become confirmed within her Church, which is part of coming to peace with herself. Caroline Ann loves to be in control of her day, her time and her own money.

Accordingly, she maps out each day for herself including where and how some support might be helpful. She reminds us that accessible, spontaneous transportation in itself would be a great support for her plans. Her days involve time for her beloved music, some assigned time for her own learning (with her new computer and math books), preparing meals, organizing her home and social life, and linking with her family and friends. She loves shopping at dollar stores and garage sales, content in the knowledge that she can control the purchases in these places. Caroline Ann completed 5 years of assisting at the Montessori school across from the co-operative, and returned to the public school nearer to her home to work. Finally Caroline Ann is fulfilled in her love for family and connection in becoming aunt to her now four-year old nephew, Terry, and keeping in close touch with her sister, Barbara.

Donna Mitchell's life has held the highest joys and the deepest sorrows over the past eight years. Four years ago, she gave birth to a beautiful baby boy, Matthew, and is realizing one of her lifelong dreams of being a mother. Matthew is a true child of Rougemount—secure, happy and loving with a wide range of people. He attends nursery school, loves balls of all kinds, is happiest when he is drawing, and insists on helping out with a range of cleaning duties in the Rougemount hallways with the cleaning staff and other co-operative members. Donna's calm nature has helped her to take on the new responsibilities of motherhood with grace and skill. Donna's mother, Marje, rejoiced in her grandson's presence since she also lived at the co-operative when he was born. To Donna's and our sorrow, Marje died in the spring of 2003. Donna and Matthew miss her greatly. We believe Donna's circle was greatly strengthened four years ago when it prepared to help Donna welcome Matthew to the world and committed to help her through. This strength has been successfully tested over the past year as circle members have managed to figure out finances, budgets, Supporter invoices, important celebrations, holidays and more. Despite their sadness, Donna and Matthew have found many wonderful times with good friends and family over the past year.

John Hobson has a full and busy life, which is centred around his family on weekends, and around his friends at *Kathryn's Restaurant* next door all other days of the week. John is involved with many family members of his own as well as Jeany's (father's partner) family. Family times together involve people of several generations, travel, fixing up the family cottage, sports events, and many celebrations. At other times, and also during the weekend if time permits, John finds time to spend with his friends at *Kathryn's*. He helps out in a number of ways at the busy restaurant. In return, he enjoys hanging out with the staff at quiet times, being the keeper of the remote control for the television in the sports bar, pulling himself fountain drinks and even beginning to learn to serve a few tables. Most of all, at *Kathryn's,* John has found a good place to hang out where he is welcomed, appreciated, accepted and where he really belongs. Other parts of John's weeks are filled with a part time job at Burger King, John's keen interest in following the Toronto Maple Leafs or Montreal Expo games (depending on the season) and keeping track of the Oshawa Generals hockey team.

Jon Bennett had started a small, portable shredding business (*J.B. Shredding*) some time ago, and in the last two years it has really taken off. He has several paying customers at this point, and also some customers who want his shredded material at the end of the day. He has moved from being a simple hand shredder to alternating this with a small portable shredding machine. Being a small business owner and spending some of his earnings makes up an important part of Jon's week. He has experimented with some very practical calendar and planning systems to help him gain greater control of his days and weeks, and is working well now with a digital-photo system that looks very high tech indeed. Jon has travelled much over the past few years: Ireland, Florida and to several places in Ontario. Jon spends time with his sister, his two aunts and his grandmother whenever he can. In his co-operative apartment, Jon celebrates each passing holiday with passion and co-operative neighbours have come to look forward to checking out his elaborate apartment decorations each time. Jon uses the internet for the exploration of his favourite topics: scary movies, haunted houses, anything undersea, Florida, and Halloween.

Rob Salmers spends his days out and about in many places and in many ways in his community. We are constantly reminded of his popularity by the number of people who greet him and know him along the Pickering streets. In addition, Rob's parents often bump into still more people who speak of talking to him recently in this or that location. Rob is a regular fan of the Ajax Community Orchestra and is a faithful audience at their Wednesday practices. He is welcomed at his local library where the librarian keeps a warm seat near the fireplace free for him on winter days. He is a swimmer who swims at least twice a week with a group of older men, a volunteer who helps out every week in the nursing home where his grandmother lives, and then again at a wildlife park. He has just starting going to a local church. *Rob's Small Parcel Delivery* is a courier business that Rob started about five years ago. There have been ups and downs in profit margins, but Rob's circle seems to find ways to regenerate business when necessary. Rob has good connections in his co-operative home as well. Last year, a spring tea brought over 35 family and friends together for a lovely afternoon.

Tiffany Dawe is fully exploring the role of artist. With the support of fellow-artist Diane Huson, she has created a growing number of beautiful watercolour paintings. She has become a member of a local art guild, and has participated in one juried art show and several other exhibitions. Tiffany has persevered as a gardener of the Rouge Valley Butterfly Garden, affording us many opportunities for learning. Her devotion has paid off by allowing her to move into a variety of office volunteer roles within the Pearce House offices throughout the winter, so that her involvement is now year round. Tiffany continues a deep and loving relationship with her half-brother, David, now five years old, and is proud first-time aunt to Britney. Her *The Tiffany Touch* baking business that she developed 9 years ago is at a low ebb. Although the demand is there, we are unable to make this a profitable proposition without an infusion of money to support expansion. She continues to run it as a very low profile business for the time being. We continue to uphold Tiffany's long term dream of establishing a co-operative tea-room meeting place for people to gather, have a cup of tea, and enjoy or purchase a variety of art that will surround them.

As for the board of Deohaeko, all of whom are family members, time has not stood still.

The Families

All of the families are eight years older than the end of the last book, and 15 years older than they were at the beginning of the Deohaeko story. It will not be surprising to hear that health issues, tiredness, and feeling the squeeze between their own parents who need their help and their children (and not just these ones!) who need support are major issues for all families. The past eight years have included early retirement forced by poor health, several hospitalizations, and several parents with new health conditions to monitor and treat.

At the same time, people continue to make important decisions about the roles and tasks that they will continue to take on despite other pressures. This group of families continue to play vital community and leadership roles in Durham Region and beyond. Some of the parents sit on other community boards. Others do presentations for family groups, small organizations and conferences across Ontario and beyond. All parents spend some of their time hosting visitors and explaining Deohaeko and our thinking to college students, foreign exchange students, families who travel in for a visit, and those who stay a bit longer. Many family members are recognized leaders in our community on issues of planning, individualized funding, circles of support, and ensuring a good life for people with a disability. These people are called in to talk with families, attend committees, and join meeting to struggle with new issues. Many of the parents work full or part time in other fields altogether. Several parents are involved with local service organizations. All parents are present throughout the week bringing ideas, strategies and a helping hand to the whole of the co-operative community. New limitations on health and energy are factors to take into consideration, but are by no means deterrents to the work that needs to be done.

Life has many good times in other ways, too. Most family members have taken on new roles as grandparents and delight in this time, while wishing they had more time to enjoy this phase in life. Helen and George welcome Terry. Linda welcomes Britney and David, Tiffany's half-brother. Elizabeth finds time for Matthew, Cameron and Jillian in addition to the three she had before. Harriet and Orest spend time with their five grandchildren. Margaret and Hilda welcome little Sam. Marje doted on Matthew, her fifth grandchild who was a special joy because he lived just one floor below her at Rougemount. Doug has linked up with a new partner, Jeany, and a whole new extended family.

Pam Hazeltine, president for many years, and friend to all the families, died in the October of 1999. Her calm presence is greatly missed by the remaining families. Her daughter, Ann, continues to live in Orangeville amid familiar friends and support people. She visits her father (Pam's husband, Walter, died 2005) and sisters at home regularly. Now Ann and her sister, Sandra are the regular family representatives at Deohaeko celebrations.

Margaret Presutti's husband, Sam died in the Spring of 2001. While not directly involved in Deohaeko Support Network, he generously shared Margaret's time with us so that we could benefit from her energy, ideas and presence. We are grateful for Margaret's, and her mother Hilda's, continued work in board and many other roles.

In March of 2003, our dear friend, fellow collaborator, and ally, Marjorie Mitchell died after a short intense illness. This has perhaps been the most serious blow to us so far—a call to remind us of the importance of our path. For the first time, one of our children is left without parents. In the last chapter, we will discuss what this has come to mean for our group.

Deohaeko Support Network

Deohaeko Support Network now consists of seven supported individuals and their families, plus the Presutti family (daughter, Corinne died in 1991), who remain active with the board, and the Hazeltine family.

Three families left over the past six years for a variety of reasons, although each reason boiled down to a disagreement over the basic principles which the families had formulated over hours of discussion. Although Deohaeko Support Network families were saddened by each of these departures, there was also a sense of understanding that came with each situation. Each situation was preceded by a period of tension and then a slow realization that things were not going to work out. Two of the supported individuals continued to make Rougemount their home for many years after their families left Deohaeko formally and they continued to benefit from the informal supports that all families worked together to make possible in the early days of Rougemount. Another individual lives with her family not far away and maintains contact with a couple of the Deohaeko families.

In each of these situations, the end of the tension was a relief. The sense of being able to get back to the matters that concerned them most—the building of good lives for their sons and daughters, rather than uncomfortable disagreements over principles that clearly could not be resolved—was most welcomed by the remaining families. At the same time, the group is greatly strengthened by the discussions involved in each leave-taking. Important priorities and principles were established and underscored among the remaining eight families (seven with a son or daughter to support).

Supportive others, including circle members, other family members, relatives, and paid Supporters also play an important role within Deohaeko Support Network. The relationships that surround and support us everyday remind us of the joy and richness of living interwoven lives.

Rougemount Housing Co-operative

There have been some important changes within Rougemount that have affected the Deohaeko Support Network families.

Over housing: For six years, the families of people who required support during the night grappled with the co-operative's issues with 'over housing' (deemed to have too many bedrooms for the number of people living in the unit). In the situations where typical roommates were desired and recruited there were no problems. In that way, a two-bedroom apartment had two occupants and the co-operative and the Ministry felt that it was meeting its accommodation commitment to the community.

However, for a few individuals, a second bedroom was necessary for an overnight support person on a temporary or permanent basis. Since this overnight person had their own home, they did not qualify as someone requiring accommodation and therefore the individuals in these two bedroom apartments were deemed to be 'over housed'.

Moving to one-bedroom units caused all kinds of problems. It was clearly very crowded and lacking in basic privacy to have the overnight person sleep on the living room sofa. The individual who lived in the apartment and was a member of the co-operative could not freely use their apartment as they might wish when there was a support person asleep in their living room. Also, one person had tried out several roommates and did not find a good fit. Her mother felt sure that we would find the right kind of situation over time, or that always leaving that as an option was important to her daughter's safety and security. By the time it was suggested that the daughter was over housed, she had been living in that unit for six years, since the opening of the co-operative. To her, this was home. We felt it was necessary for the person's sense of home to remain in their apartment despite changing support requirements. We felt and argued that the Ministry was meeting its accommodation goals by providing access to affordable housing to people who might not otherwise be able to live in their own homes.

This issue was discussed at some length with the board and Rougemount members for several years. We always had a good level of support and understanding from co-operative members. The board in its role to represent all of the community was only cautious that all members were afforded the same opportunities. In the end, in December of 2000, we met with Ministry officials who understood the concept immediately and the longstanding over housing issue was resolved. We were overjoyed. This meant long-term security for at least three or four people right away. It offered a way to look at accommodation that was centred on the supports a person may require, not the special status of Deohaeko members. This understanding could affect any Rougemount member should the time come when they required such support.

In 2002, the provincial government saw fit to 'download' housing co-operatives from provincial government responsibility and control to the local regional government. We are told that our hard won understanding on the part of the Ministry will no longer necessarily be acceptable to the local Region. Here we go again! This is the first rule of community—it is never really over. We win many struggles and enjoy our periods of peace and growth, but the need for vigilance is constant. We may well have to come back to this same struggle once again.

Rougemount board membership: Another significant change that has affected the Deohaeko-Rougemount relationship was the Rougemount board decision in the Spring of 2002 that Rougemount was acting outside of its legal bylaws in reserving two board seats for Deohaeko members. While this was strictly true, this practice had been supported by the membership for six years after a vote at a General Members' Meeting. There had never been any dissent to the decision, and other boards had always seemed to welcome our experience, commitment and sense of history and vision. It was well known that it would only take a small legal change in the by-law to make this practice legal. At the time, this change was not done for political reasons—no other co-operative had this status yet, and our community was so supportive that it was seen as unnecessary. Typically, Deohaeko members at the Rougemount board filled many welcomed roles. They provided continuity and a sense of history for new board members. They had many years of board experience and could act as models and guides to new board members when they started their terms. The encouragement of the intentional community was uppermost in their minds (not just representing the interests of their own son or daughter) and so they brought a broader picture to the board. They were skilled and committed to consensus-building and helping others to grow in their roles. They were unflagging committee members and could be found at the heart of most social and work-party gatherings. They knew most members and could represent many people who exercised little voice in the community.

This Rougemount board decision clearly came from other roots and was at first a blow to Deohaeko and the way it saw its role in protecting and encouraging intentional community. Despite many members' interest and work, this decision remained unchanged. Members passed motions at General Members' Meetings to have the legal work done to reverse this decision, but to this day no further progress has been made. Clearly, there were political forces influencing board decisions over which we had no control.

Meanwhile, Deohaeko members decided that we had more than enough work to do without bemoaning the loss of one more board commitment. We believed that our role could still be played out in the typical community, and set about continuing our vital part of community. There is a change in the community, to be sure. However, the foundations remain strong and Rougemount remains to provide many safe, welcoming opportunities for the sons and daughters of the founding members.

Moving to a project management team: Hiring an independent staff team to manage the co-operative (co-operative coordinator, administrative assistant, community facilitator, and maintenance crew) directed by the board of directors was a model that worked well for the first seven years for Rougemount. However, when problems arose they arose quickly and deeply and the inexperienced board at the time was convinced to move to an external management team model within the co-operative. This has only been in place for less than a year, but there are reservations within the community about the effectiveness of this model. Individual staff answerable to the board seemed much more open to learning about how this particular community wanted to live its intentional community spirit. A project management team is mystified by this desire for one of its project sites to do things differently than the others. Only time will tell how this particular dynamic will play itself out. Once again, we need to exercise vigilance and seize every opportunity to do things in our own way. That is the role that Deohaeko has taken on from the very beginning—to be the flame that calls people back to our original intentions for an inclusive, welcoming community.

These events were perhaps the beginning of raising our awareness about the need to safeguard some aspects of our lives and work. People's homes were threatened with over housing issues, the quality of the intentional community was jeopardized by a small but effective faction that questioned Deohaeko's presence at the board level. At the same time, as we will discuss elsewhere, we became aware of various movements all through the greater community that could serve to threaten or alienate its most vulnerable members, including our sons and daughters. We began to realize that a much more conscious effort to vigilance and awareness would be needed. We talk more about the issue of safeguarding in Chapter 9.

Within Deohaeko—Where Do We Put Our Energy?

Within Deohaeko itself, we have much to keep us busy. Issues in the broader community and in the Rougemount community are part of the framework in which we live and work. But we also focus our thoughts and efforts one by one on each individual and family within our own context.

a) **Articulating our principles** was a major focus for several years. Then we went through a period of feeling that we were smaller, and it was obvious that we were a more cohesive group. We felt less of a need to write these down. Lately however, we have a our growing awareness that someone must always be as vigilant as we try to be, and that people who take on a lead role for our sons and daughters in the future might benefit from some written assistance. Now, we are through completing a rich, clear written document that we intend to continue to work on, but which will provide direction for other family members, circle members and Supporters for years to come. Our annual two-day retreats are a constant source of renewal, focus and planning for us. It remains our chance to step back and decide on our reactions to the events around us. Chapter 2 outlines our work so far on principles.

b) **Circles** are still a key way to help us think about relationship. We spend time building circles, expanding them, worrying about their content, their membership, their frequency, and their relevance. We are perhaps more aware than ever of the importance of lively, committed circles. We are not there yet and our road is bumpy and imperfect. We believe that circles of committed people, who know our son or daughter in a personal way over time, are the best assurance for a positive future. In an effective circle each individual knows the person in some way, but no one person feels the overwhelming responsibility to know or take charge of all of the areas at once. Some of our circles are beginning to look a bit like this. Over time, some parents have been persuaded to let go a little bit and share some of the work in some circles. There are more details about our struggles here in Chapter 4.

c) The issue of **Supporters** always gives us lots to think about. Good Supporters are hard to find, complicated to guide, and difficult to keep. We continue to explore new ways of finding people, scheduling, and guiding them. In the middle of all of the struggles, we celebrate the presence of six Supporters who have been with us for more than five years. More about this in Chapter 8.

d) Deohaeko Support Network continues with **one main coordinator** (myself) who has now been with the families for over ten years. There have been benefits to this consistency to Deohaeko, to the families, and to the individuals (as well as to me). There has been a consistent agenda of the work to be done and where we are headed. We have not had to use up valuable time in regular orientation of new coordinators. We know each other well and know how to work together. When there are conflicts, we work them through. We rely on each other. In some areas, we can really deepen the work. At the same time, we worry about the future. How do we think about coordinators for the future? What new sets of skills and ideas might be more helpful for the challenges ahead? How do we find good coordinators? How do we help them learn? The role of our coordinator is discussed in detail in Chapter 8.

e) **Funding from government source**s has not changed much in the past eight years. Our annualized funding which became firm in 1996 has remained constant except for portions given up as individual families have left Deohaeko. In September 1999 we began to run a weekly Sunday morning Bingo. This enables us to meet our annual deficit, although we are well aware that this is a short term solution to a long term problem. We continue to look for ways to let the government know that its funds do not currently meet our support requirements. See Chapter 10 for more on money matters.

f) In December 1999 we were delighted to learn that we had received our 5-Year Ontario **Trillium Foundation grant**, *Our Presence Has Roots*. We are currently in Year 5 of this project and it is enabling us to investigate and implement ways to sustain the presence and gifts of our sons and daughters in the community over time. The project is a two-fold attempt to research and meet both the financial security needs of people and the need to live meaningful lives rooted in community roles among people who know them personally and have some commitment to their future. This book is the outcome of the work on learning about community connections and relationships. Another book, *On Our Own...Together* (2002), researched and written by Harry van Bommel addresses the financial security elements, namely trust funds for financially-dependent loved ones and endowment funds for charitable organizations like our own. It was distributed free of charge to over 1100 families and organizations across Canada in 2002.

g) In June 2002, after two and a half years of time-consuming research, much discussion among families and a lot of hard, hard work, Deohaeko Support Network signed an **Endowment** agreement with the Community Foundation of Durham Region. Although a major step in itself, the challenge of filling this endowment fund to meaningful levels remains to be met.

Deohaeko—Looking Outward

Right at the start, Deohaeko made a commitment to support other like-minded families not by expanding but by providing information to families and opportunities to dream for themselves. In the past six years Deohaeko members have met families in many places: in living rooms and coffee shops, at circle meetings, by presenting at local Association meetings, taking part in other Trillium projects to inform families of new ways of doing things, at local and international conferences, at local community colleges, by linking with university research projects, and at a myriad of social role valorization-based workshops and gatherings. In particular, our parents, Linda Dawe and Helen Dionne, have become names that other families recognize instantly as expert and reliable resources for thoughtful discussions about family support, finding a home, and co-operative living options.

In the Durham Region of Ontario where Deohaeko has its heart, there are an unusually large number of family groups—groups of families who join together to find a suitable and sustaining way to support their sons and daughters to live a full life within the communities of their choosing. This phenomenon is due in no small part to Peter Dill, during many of these years, but no longer, Executive Director of the Ajax-Pickering-Whitby Association for Community Living. He acted on his commitment early in his life to "act in such a way as to be with people where they are, to listen deeply and to invite others, because of what I learned from Jean Vanier and Wolf Wolfensberger that it is out of the personal relationship that things happen". We keep in touch with the other family groups on matters that concern us all: Supporters, learning opportunities, common values, community connections.

Deohaeko families are also very active with a small informal group of like-minded people who gather at Rougemount every second Friday. This group of families, professionals, interested individuals, and common allies comes together to discuss and engage in the work that we have been called to do—building healthy communities and safeguarding the work of including the gifts and presence of people who are the most vulnerable. This group is like a nutrient-rich dose of sustenance to many of us every other week. It allows us to know that we have supportive colleagues and allies every step we take.

Chapter 2
Philosophy at the Foundation

We began our journey more than a decade ago with a simple, yet practical set of concepts that served to guide our earliest plans, dreams, proposal-writing, and decisions. We said that we followed a philosophy that honoured five principles:

1. Individualization
2. Social Support
3. Self-Determination
4. Participation
5. Non-Discrimination

Looking back at these five guiding concepts, I am struck with how the words might have meant very different things for other people. Even with our accompanying explanations, these very same descriptions might have led to very different responses. For us, over time, it is very clear that it was our ongoing dialogues with each other, our constant clarification, and our determined late night discussions that led us to finding these few words to be helpful and directive. What we now know is that *nothing* can replace talking with each other, and listening deeply and openly to responses that are different from our own.

Over the years, we began to realize how important it was to share with significant others the common understandings we grew to have with each other. We understood that our actions were based on a common way of believing and thinking about the world. If we want others who will have an impact on the lives of our sons and daughters (sisters and brothers, other relatives, circle members) to continue with similar actions and decisions, they must come from a common way of understanding the world.

Perhaps because we were dealing with many people who did not have the time or commitment to enter into a full study of these simple principles, we used very concrete and practical ways of describing our beliefs and intentions. These included a series of statements with a principled component followed by a practical component that directed people to right action.

This person is a unique individual whose life has value and purpose—just like any other person in our community. Therefore her uniqueness is to be discovered, her gifts are to be recognized, her time is to be well spent in interesting and meaningful ways, and her presence is to be celebrated. Each person's lives, plans, goals and aspirations are different. Let this be your guide.

This person is able to contribute to her community in meaningful ways. Community is stronger and healthier when the gifts and contributions of all members in community life are welcomed. Everyone benefits by taking part in an inclusive, welcoming community life.

This person shares in all of the rights, privileges, and responsibilities of adult citizens of this community. Therefore, no exceptions need be made on the basis of disability. We can creatively design, accommodate and discover ways to make this all possible.

This person can and does essentially govern her own life. At the same time, this person needs the ongoing, thoughtful consideration of her family and a few others (her circle) in order to ensure that her voice is heard, her dreams are brought into being, her responsibilities are met, her gifts are recognized and cherished, and her support requirements are met.

This person shares in the interests, dreams, and choices of her age peers. Therefore, with support and accommodation, there is little she cannot do or explore.

Her range of options and choices should be typical of other people of her age and gender in her community.

This person has the interest and ability to be involved in enduring personal relationships and requires ample opportunity to do so. The development of healthy, mutual and enduring relationships of various kinds is the primary focus of our work. We believe that this can primarily occur in highly valued, typical settings in the presence of typical citizens of Durham Region. Therefore, settings and situations which other citizens typically choose are preferable to segregated options.

The gifts and possibilities inherent in natural, informal relationships give these preference over formal, paid relationships. Therefore, a Supporter's ultimate goal is to provide support in such a way that over the long run the individual meets and develops a variety of relationships with other people who are not paid to be with them.

We need to acknowledge the uniqueness of each individual, while understanding that our strength comes from working together as a group. Deohaeko came together as a group that shares common vision and values, including the belief that by working together, we are stronger and more able to achieve our vision. At the same time, its membership is essentially one of individuals, and we seek to work in ways which underline the uniqueness and individuality of each family and their son or daughter. Therefore, funding is requested on an individual basis, funds received are allocated on an individual basis naturally leading to Supporters being hired by one family at a time, and each person's life and plans are very different. General guidelines outline our common approach, but family may make an alternate decision based on their unique experience within the context of our principles.

Our work is about changing the world. We are challenging the status quo. We are modelling another way. We are trying to discover new ways (or re-discover old ways) for people to relate to one another by focusing on gifts and possibilities, rather than deficits and limitations. We need to look for this in the arrangements that surround our sons and daughters, but also we need to model this in all of our dealings within the community and the rest of the world. This means that our work may be difficult, poorly understood or accepted, and constantly threatened. This also means that our efforts make a difference in individual lives, one person at a time.

We have found this set of statements to be practical and useful in helping new Supporters, circle members and various others become more skilled and adept at making value-based decisions and choices in the presence of our family member. They seemed to touch on all of the important values that we held—value of the individual, emphasis on similarities with age-gender peers, valued social roles, and relationship.

In speaking with families in all parts of this province, and sometimes farther afield, Linda Dawe and I find it useful to focus on a group of principles that seem to comprise the most important elements of our thinking. Oral presentations do not often allow for time to fully describe important foundational thinking which underpin one's work. This list of statements is a brief list of core beliefs. This became one way of helping others understand that our way of thinking and acting does not just come 'from the gut' but rather is built on something more solid, systematic and explicit. We usually describe them as follows:

- Every person has value.
- People are individuals. Everyone's lives, plans, goals and aspirations are different. This is what always guides us.

- In the end, it is people who make a difference in our lives.
- We must, in everything we do, focus on relationships.
- Everyone is able to contribute. Period!
- We need to ensure that everyone has the opportunity to contribute because this is what is best for the whole community.
- In order to plan and think things through and to achieve what is best, we must always look to what is typical for people of the same age and gender who live good lives in our community.

These strategies worked well for us in the beginning years when we were younger, healthier and more firmly in control of what others thought and did even when not in our presence. The last eight years have been years where the limits of our personal presence now and in the future are becoming all too obvious. We are starting to meet the very real limits of our physical capacity to keep on top of all decisions and directions. We are also more aware than ever before of the complexity of the world around us and the constant challenges to our vulnerable family members. It is simply harder to make quick decisions. We no longer have the same faith in the sufficiency of our earlier, simple words or our practical definitions of how to make decisions. They do not seem to be adequate for the purposes of those who come after—too much is left up in the air.

We knew that there were complexities, dangers, and shortcomings in our practical, word-of-mouth approach of the past to making sure that the lives of our loved ones continue to move in positive directions. The paths to resolving inevitable conflicts and differing perceptions are fraught with danger. A way of easing the danger seemed to be in preparing a written foundation that people in the future could return to for making all kinds of decisions. We knew that there are many situations in which the best or 'right' decision is not obvious. We wanted to raise awareness of these 'danger' situations as a reminder to ourselves and as guideposts for future generations of co-decision makers.

Typical dangers that we encounter and expect that others will encounter in the future are described here in some detail.

One danger is the exception. You are asked to make a decision that you would not ordinarily make, usually due to unusual circumstances. "We'll just make this one exception. We'll just do it this time. It's okay, it is an emergency." Occasionally, this is true. More often, five minutes in that direction renders us incapable of thinking of better alternatives. And once no better alternatives can be found during this exception, then all such situations will result in the exception. Quickly, the exception becomes the norm. How to decide if this exception might be safe and revocable? We needed a higher level set of principles and beliefs against which people can gauge whether they are talking about lower level practicalities that might be set aside and easily regained, or one of our most basic principles.

For example, Brenda's mother is stuck in traffic and cannot meet up with Brenda for tea as planned. She asks if Brenda might go to Tiffany's for tea so that she will not be alone while her mother makes her way through traffic. As a one-time event, Brenda and Tiffany *would* enjoy tea together and this would be a safer alternative than Brenda being on her own. This may be an acceptable exception to our principle of not grouping people together for support and one that is easily limited to one time. On the other hand, according to our belief in the utmost importance of relationship, an even better alternative might be an opportunity for Brenda to spend an hour with another neighbour, where both could benefit from spending some time together. Either way, however, might be acceptable one-time decisions.

However, future planners in Brenda's circle may come together at some point to think about how Brenda might best spend her tea times (which are very important to her) during all of the week days. Our principles would let them know that daily tea times with Tiffany are not an acceptable way to think about or plan for Brenda's time. On a frequent and regular basis, this would put one Supporter in the position of supporting two people. It would group people for support, and most importantly these outcomes would greatly impede any possibility of Brenda moving into relationship with other neighbours in her co-operative. With thought and support, tea time is a great opportunity for Brenda to have a deeper relationship with one or more of her other neighbours.

Another danger is "but there are no other funds". People are often asked to share or make do with less than adequate funding. This often causes people to panic and grab onto whatever little bit of resource they can—even without examining whether or not it comes with unacceptable conditions. We needed some ways of thinking for ourselves and others later on that would guide us in deciding which conditions would be unacceptable. For example, we had already set in place practices that meant that no two people would receive support from the same Supporter at the same time (e.g., always 1:1 support). This belief led us to very creative alternatives to paid support. These range from short visits from and with friends and neighbours, greater involvement of parents and other family members, experimenting with short periods of unsupervised leisure time, and using natural supports within work, volunteer and recreational sites. We needed to develop a way to describe the world that we wanted for ourselves and our loved ones and the many alternates ways of getting there.

A further danger is "well, she likes it—or it's her choice". On the face of it, this seems to be a simple opportunity to support a person's autonomy. However, if the choice is one that will not reflect very positively on her image, her health, her skills, or her life in general, we know that such situations demand a more respectful and careful reaction. It is important to understand whether this is the informed decision of someone that has explored and experienced the alternatives, or whether it is the weary defiance of being offered two or fewer unsatisfactory options. If it truly is her choice, the question becomes how to make it as safe and valued as possible. This decision has many possible outcomes. We needed ways of helping future generations figure this out.

Another danger is "settling for less". We see that John has a good life compared to other young men with disabilities that his family knows, or compared to five years ago when we were just starting out. We feel that we should be grateful for these gains, and we can rest on our laurels that all is well. None of the reigning principles is obviously broken, and there are few problems to face. We needed words and ideas that would inspire ourselves, circle members and future board members to challenge complacency and 'good enough'. We had come to know that rarely is anything 'static' and doing nothing usually meant that things are sliding backwards. We had also come to understand the nature of our children's vulnerabilities is such that settling for less is always damaging. Besides, when has anything but the best and ongoing efforts been good enough for anyone's children? These were thoughts that we wanted to leave for members of the future.

A final and constant danger arises when, despite our best efforts, we do not have a resolution at hand that seems to work in difficult situations. These situations are especially ones involving emotional and distraught individuals, medical problems that loom uncertainly, or habits and behaviour patterns that constantly go against generally-agreed upon norms of society. A very typical response by other well-meaning family members or circle members when faced with difficult issues, is to turn to the disability service system as a last-ditch option. We needed a statement that would have circle members and others who take on an accompanying role with people to understand that *we are the option of choice.*

When all seems to fail, and things are not going according to plan, we are still the best option. Certainly, there are such times when our plans need serious reconsideration. We might have to try very different alternatives. However, what we have to offer is not provided anywhere else. Each one of our circles provides a group of people who know the individual well over a longer period of time. They have known him through other difficult times, and they also know what he is like when life is good for him. Even more importantly, they care for him and about what happens to him. Even in the worst crisis, better that this group of caring, creative people make plans and decisions about a person they know, than a service or organization looking to provide for another client, in a model based on group care and group approaches. Our alternatives based on love, caring and knowing the person intimately are the best option to provide people with what they really need and want. We will gather resources, gain skills, find the right people and not give up until we have a workable solution. We needed this to be written so that others would have a chance to discuss this and hopefully begin to feel the same resolve.

Due to the limits of our health and energy, and the extreme complexities of the world around us, we have started to contemplate those who will come after us and what will guide them. We understand more fully than ever before that we will not always be here. We understand that good decisions are harder to make in today's world. We understand that how we view our family members and our way of seeing community life are not typical ways that most people in today's society see these things. We needed a place to begin to articulate our unique and powerful vision of our world.

And so, very slowly over a period of eight years we have tried to put on paper that which is already written in our hearts and minds. We have tried to find the words, thoughts, and beliefs that inspire us, in the hope that they will also inspire others. We have tried to foresee the most typical or difficult situations and make a special address to that. We have tried to keep in mind our view for the whole community, not just for our family or family member, because embedded in it all is the belief that what is good for our family member will be good for the entire community. That is the gift of our son or daughter.

We have stopped and started many times, because often we know that words alone will not do the job. We have to prepare the hearts and minds of those who will one day receive the words. We need to spend time working on family relationships so that the relationship is firm and deep, and the words will make some sense. We need to figure out how to provide opportunities for the others to think and talk and listen, just as we ourselves have done. So, our progress is slow. What you see here is only the written part—not the anguish and the questioning and the re-building of sibling relationships and the efforts to provide forums of deep discussion.

In many ways we are reluctant to present the document of our principles here for all the world to see. We know that people can be taken away by pretty words and believe that they alone might mean something. We know that this is a work in progress for us, and what we write today will be amended somewhat in word or nuance by our experiences tomorrow.

At the same time, when we came to write the principles document, we found it very difficult to find other models to follow. We knew that we wanted to examine some pretty fundamental beliefs but we found it hard to find a list of what these might be. We knew the pieces of a document that we wanted to come together, but we were at a loss for a format that would help us lay it out. So, in honour of those who intend to do just as much talking, thinking and praying as we have over their own sets of beliefs and principles, we offer you our efforts as one model for you to consider. Don't copy it—create your own, but learn from our efforts, too.

How Principles Arise Directly Out of Our Experience

A reproduction of our Principles document in this book would simply be a dry copy of what is a living document for us because we live it and work with it every day. Instead, in an attempt to provide something more widely useful, I will spend some time looking at some of the significant experiences that led us to include certain sections or statements within our document. *Please note that sections copied directly from our Principles Document are written in italics.*

Choosing Our Own Way

An early common experience among the families was the recognition that our family members with disabilities are not valued in our present-day society. Once we were able to consciously recognize that society does not value many of the qualities embodied by our family member, we are able to assert our own actions in the face of society's perceptions. In our preamble, we state that we can value people with disabilities and we can choose to do so every day.

We live in a world…

> *….where society values one set of human attributes (youth, health, conventional beauty, money, productivity, speed, intellectual accomplishment) over their opposites, and*

> *…where, in doing so, that society harms countless numbers of people, including our children with*

disabilities, who are not seen to embody the chosen attributes (people with disabilities, elderly people, and others), and

…where most people are not conscious of the impact of these values on vulnerable people, even those who care for them deeply.

We, members of Deohaeko Support Network, stand counter to the common culture and believe strongly and will act clearly to uphold our own set of principles based on the understanding that all people have intrinsic value, have gifts to share, and that our human community is better when all members share in the gifts of each other.

With this statement we remind ourselves and teach those yet to come that we are choosing another way. We choose not to devalue our sons and daughters by talking about them in complaining and negative ways. We will not and do not write 'needy' funding proposals, but rather we request funds to help them achieve typical goals and dreams. We include them as full family members because we do not believe they are a 'burden' to their brothers and sisters. We counter 'poor you' exclamations with statements of joy and appreciation for the presence of this person in our lives.

The Value and Uniqueness of Each Person

Each person is inherently worthy, a unique human being of great value. In our experience, when we truly believe this, it becomes very easy to see the importance of unique and individualized supports, plans and dreams for each person. How could the supports and dreams for any two people be the same? When we think of people very carefully one at a time, a unique and individual vision arises for each person. This is what we need to seek out and begin to put into place—not one kind of living space for all people, not one kind of day program for all people, not one kind of support person for several people.

We are all about valuing and recognizing the human quality of each and every person. This alone accords them inherent value, respect and being seen as worthy of living a good life.

We show we value each person in the following ways:

a) By ensuring that people are involved in the decisions and directions of their lives, because this leads to more meaningful decision-making and lives where people are central and have a voice.

b) By ensuring that all people have opportunities to make meaningful contributions and hold valued social roles in their communities, thereby enjoying a spirit of belonging, a sense of worth and [possibly] the respect of their community.

c) By surrounding people with high expectations of what they are capable of, how they can contribute and how they will learn and grow over their life times.

d) By allowing and supporting people to hold and meet personal responsibilities and keep commitments and promises.

e) By, even in the face of great barriers, continuing to show respect, listen deeply and be present to the person we are with.

Also, the following section reflects the uniqueness of the person.

Each family situation and each individual is unique. Getting to know our sons and daughters in an (intimate and loving) way is essential.

a) No one single answer, technique, or approach can apply to all of our sons and daughters. Each requires an individual approach, individual kinds of planning, individual funding and individual support persons.

b) Resist attempts to enter into group answers, group approaches, or design policies or rules that allow one approach, Supporter or other 'make do' for two or more people. Share ideas, learn from one another but do not replicate—none of the involved individuals will benefit.

c) It is essential that others come to know our sons and daughters in a way that is evolving over time, understanding the essence of who they are, and understanding of their life experiences and that has had an impact on their lives today.

So, this principle leads us to insist on one-to-one support for each person at all times. This means that at all times that support is in place, the person gets the unique and individualized attention that works best for them.

Individual wishes, demands and support requirements simply cannot be met with anything less than the full attention of one supportive person at a time. Individual gifts, talents and skills cannot be highlighted when support is to be shared with another, equally unique but differently gifted person who requires support. Where you go, what you do, how you do it and how you interact with the other people with whom you come into contact will be severely compromised when there is anything less than one-to-one support.

Secondly, this principle has led us to decide that Supporters are not shared among families. Each individual requires support in a different way, with different skills, at different times and with a certain amount of flexibility. We know that this cannot happen for two families at one time. It is hard to imagine one person fitting well with two very unique situations. As well, one Supporter working with more than one family can develop a 'caseload' mentality which is the antithesis of our focus on the individual. There are inevitably conflicts in times of support, circle gatherings, and other factors. Each family offers a different work environment and different communication styles and a Supporter might naturally fit with one better than another. This leads to dissent among the families. Unity within a family group is very important and worth extra effort to preserve.

Thirdly, this principle with its focus on uniqueness leads us to understand that people need to live in their own homes and not share then with another vulnerable person who has their set of unique support requirements. It is very difficult to make one living space feel truly like home to two or more vulnerable people who would have different requirements for noise, quiet, structure, routine, support, and space, not to mention tastes in décor, music, and social standards. This principle arises directly out of our experience. In the early days, there were two situations where two individuals were to share their home. The longest lasted a few weeks before the urge to support each person fully and uniquely led us to design very separate homes for each of them.

Valuing Community

We have come to a deeper understanding of the riches and the safeguards inherent in community and we found ways to include this in our document.

Community is stronger and healthier when we find ways to make room for supporting and safeguarding the presence of all members of the community within the community.

Therefore, we are about:

a) Helping people to come together and to get to know one another in genuine ways because people benefit from their relationships with other people and all people need opportunities to both give and receive of one another.

b) Promoting community life over its segregating alternatives. Human relationships and community are highly complex social entities where many things are possible and both good and bad can happen. Alternatives to true community (which are by definition not visible to the typical citizen) provide much greater risks to the well being of vulnerable people, and none of its rich potential.

People may need protection or safeguarding in community, but it is relationships that really keep a person safe. It is only in community—among typical, valued people—that people are truly safe. Not in services. Not in programs. Not apart from what is deemed proper and good for the rest of our community.

c) Acting on the understanding that life is better for our sons and daughters when they are present and contributing members of their community.

Participating means being a part of and knowing other people. This makes people safer. Contact with other people is a safeguard for our sons and daughters. Where there is little contact or participation, others will not know that our sons and daughters are gone and perhaps in harm. People in the community will not know to ask.

d) Avoiding temptation to turn community opportunities and the relationships therein into a commodity of our consumer-driven world. Do not let money, wages, or monetary reward drive any of your community relations. When unavoidable, let this be unintrusive, short-term, and not based on hourly rates.

For us, the latter comment has arisen from our strong convictions about not hiring people who live in the housing co-operative as Supporters. We feel that paying neighbours has the potential for destroying community for several reasons. It very powerfully undermines the message that this co-operative member is just the same as you or I. It focuses on the needs of the vulnerable person, rather than on talents, skills and similarities. It confuses people about the nature of friendship. Are you asking me to do this to get paid for it, or are you asking me to do it as a friend? How come my neighbour gets paid for this thing that you are asking me to do out of friendship? In a consumer society, it turns both members into commodities. If I get to know her will I get a job out of it? Should I pay her or should I not?

It is worth considering which community situations are close enough in nature to our co-operative situation to warrant following this directive. Might this be true for your immediate neighbourhood or for classmates in one's high school courses?

This principle also comes from our understanding of segregated events. Generally, segregated group events are harmful to both people who need support and to typical community members. Segregation of people with disabilities reinforces the already present notion in the minds and hearts of many people that people with disabilities are not like others and don't belong. This message has legitimized and led to the inhumane treatment of disabled people for many years.

We have found that a number of events do work better for us when they are limited and set apart. These include family-board retreats, learning events, and our Annual General Meeting. However, all of these events focus on the relationship with family members, friends and Supporters who do not have a disability. All other events that are segregated by disability, (e.g., planning a trip for just the sons and daughters of Deohaeko), are discouraged. We believe that if it is worthwhile doing, it is worthwhile for doing within a typical group.

We understand that people with disabilities may have genuine and fulfilling relationships with one another. Often these can be supported with minimal resources. It is not hard to do and takes minimal support skills. Often paid support is not really needed at all. We have found that our sons and daughters have ample opportunities to be around their friends and others with disabilities (as well as many occasions to be with elders and people who are very poor). What they have much less access to are thoughtful, well-supported opportunities to be genuinely involved with typical people in regular community ways.

We also know that it is safer and better (life enriching) when people are known, welcomed, accepted, and in relationship with a range of valued members of their community. However, this work is more difficult, more time-consuming, and personally riskier to do. It involves much thought, some asking, and the real possibility of rejection. There is much to learn about doing this well. If our resources and our energies are limited, let us put them here where others are not apt to do so and the outcomes are so much richer. The easier stuff will happen without us.

Relationships

The focus on much of our energy is helping our family members to develop a wide range of positive relationships in their lives. This must be seen as essential for anyone who joins us.

We are all about:

Understanding that this kind of life and community is all about relationships. We need allies, friends, and supportive others to join us in our work. We cannot do our work in isolation. We need to continually gather to us people who will stand by us and engage in the struggle.

a) We need to work continually to build bridges and support one another—by searching out, listening to, working with and supporting other like-minded families, family groups, organizations, and community associations.

b) We need to value natural relationships over paid ones. The gifts and possibilities inherent in natural, informal relationships give these preference over formal, paid relationships. Therefore, a Supporter's ultimate goal is to provide support in such a way that over the long run that support might easily and naturally be taken over by others.

Natural personal and committed relationships and good paid support are both powerful influences in the life of a person with a disability. However, these roles are not interchangeable. People do move from one to the other and there are good stories to illustrate this. These, however, are the exception. Even if people do occasionally move between the two roles, the fact remains that there are different expectations and tasks assigned to each of these roles.

An important beginning step is to visibly and verbally value natural relationships over paid ones. Teach paid Supporters to get out of the way, recognize moments of potential, support early initiatives, and take pride in being a springboard to new relationships.

Decision-Making

We have much experience in helping our family members to have a great degree of control and influence over the events of their lives. We felt it was important to put some of these into writing.

We believe that our sons and daughters ought to have input and significant control over important aspects of their lives.

a) People need the opportunity to experience the alternatives, to learn from those experiences in a positive way, and to be afforded reasonable options by those whom they trust.

b) The struggles related to ensuring that our sons and daughters are involved in making decisions in their lives in genuine ways are ongoing, complex and important.

c) Decision-making over important aspects of their lives, for our sons and daughters, should reflect the ways that other typical adults make similar decisions in their own lives—in consultation with people whom they trust and who will support them through a good decision-making process. It is also understood that government and societal rules put limits on many of our decisions and choices.

d) Choices may be offered and made at many junctures during the day and week. These may be limited or shaped by numerous structures or happenings of any given day (not enough time, persons offering support do not have the skills required, the food/choice is not currently available, too costly, etc.). At the same time, Supporters and all others providing a support role at times of possible choice must be helped to recognize the large amount of power and control that they may hold over each given opportunity to provide choice or not. They need to learn to see opportunities for offering and supporting choice, as well as to value their role in ensuring that choice and meaningful decisions are supported at every opportunity.

Setting Standards

Ensuring that people are assisted to hold typical, valued roles in their lives is linked to the expectation that people would lead lives that follow the same general balance and use of time as other people. We knew the benefits of making sure that people would have the same kinds of opportunities to enjoy life with all of its challenges and riches, just like everyone else.

We have moved through many of layers of consciousness about how to make sure that decisions made would be fully supportive of this notion. The most helpful concept that we used regularly was the imagining of a fictitious age-gender peer in Durham Region who would be a measuring stick against which we could assess our decisions.

A helpful standard for helping the individual make some important decisions about how they spend their time, money and energy is to ask: what are the valued range of responses that other highly valued people of the same age and gender would make in Durham Region?

This person shares in the interests, dreams, and choices of her age peers. Therefore, with support and accommodation, there is little she cannot do or explore. If you are wondering what to do next, ask yourself what might another person, of similar age and gender who is living a satisfying life in your area, do in her place. This usually presents you and her with a positive range of next options.

This is our day-to-day common standard. Therefore, when we felt that Jon was missing out on something in his life, we imagined (sometimes by brainstorming with other people of his age at the time) what other 21-year old men were doing with their time in Durham Region. This exercise gave us a rich range of roles and activities (work, family, learning, recreation, spiritual) from which Jon could choose how he might want to spend his time. When we were trying to think about how to help Donna with her grief over the death of her mother, we turned to our own experiences and those of other younger people in the area. We turned away from grief programs and groups and into many, many opportunities to talk, reminisce and cry with friends, and a few organized community events for friends to join and reminisce together.

The Good Life

The idea of a high standard based in typical, valued community life led us to think about our own general ideas of what it is to live a meaningful life.

We want this person's life to contain the same things that all of us would include to describe a good and meaningful life:

- *A place to call home.*
- *Safety and security in one's home and wherever they go in their community and wider abroad.*
- *Connections to family, friends, and a wide range of acquaintances—people who value them for their own unique combination of character, gifts, talents, and strengths.*

- *A sense of belonging—people who value their presence and miss her when she is not present.*
- *A place of places to give, participate, and contribute in meaningful ways that are recognized, appreciated and welcomed.*
- *Spending their days in personally fulfilling ways.*
- *Continual opportunities to grow and expectations that they will grown and learn throughout their lifetime.*
- *Respect of those with whom they come into contact.*
- *The opportunity to make good, well-supported choices and to be involved with governing the direction of their life.*
- *Good health as a result of living a healthy life style.*
- *A few close and committed relationships with family members and friends, and an ever-widening circle of those committed to be with them on their life's journey.*
- *A way to communicate with at least a small circle of people who understand them well and care to listen to the deeper messages within actions and responses to situations.*
- *Hope for the future.*
- *The opportunity to work on a few of life's dreams at any given time.*
- *A satisfying spiritual life.*

All decisions made for and with our sons and daughters should be based on ensuring that at least one or more of these elements are met.

These Things Make a Day Complete

We thought about what would constitute a good day for ourselves, as valued citizens. We felt strongly that our family member would certainly enjoy no less of a list than this for their own experience of a good day.

These are the things that make a day complete:
- *Starting and ending the day in your own home.*
- *Including a range of other people in your day.*

- *Having an opportunity to invite someone in some way.*
- *Having a chance to contribute.*
- *Exploring something new or old.*
- *Knowing that someone cares about you, and caring for someone else.*
- *Having some time to oneself.*
- *Being busy, if one chooses.*
- *Being involved in the mundane, everyday things in life.*
- *Learning something.*
- *Enjoying food that keeps you well.*
- *Having exercise and fresh air in ways that feel just right.*
- *Being reminded that you belong.*
- *Having a chance to recreate or follow a leisure pursuit.*
- *Having an impact—directing something, making a difference.*
- *Taking responsibility.*

Having written the list, and understanding its importance, we strive to make all of these things an everyday part of the experience of how our family members spend their time. They are simple things in many ways, but they have made a big difference.

Starting and ending the day in your own home has meant for us that people begin and end their days in rhythms that are unique and meaningful to them. They do not all get up at the same time and go to day programs which then fill their day. Instead, people begin their days at home by getting up and ready for the day in ways that are uniquely suited to them. Some people get up early and leave their homes right away. Some people sleep in and move into their day at a leisurely pace. People move into whatever has been deemed as of interest and value to the individual as guided by family and circle. Some people move into work situations. Some people volunteer in their community.

Some people manage their home and other affairs. Some people pursue leisure interests. Some people work at their own businesses.

In the same way, the end of the day is typically in their own homes, with evening routines and rituals that lead to a good sleep in their own beds. This sounds very simple and it is, but in the beginning it takes a lot of effort to say 'no' to other ways about thinking of one's time. We had to realize that while a day program might fill a day, it could never meet the unique and ever-changing aspirations of our family members. We realized how much we had been conditioned to thinking about a day program to provide for work or leisure for our family members with a disability. Instead, we began to think about and take responsibility for all of the events and activities that might fill a unique and meaningful day for and with each person.

Once you begin to think of assisting people to include a range of people in their day, it is easier to think about getting out of one's home at some point and being in places where one is apt to meet other people. It also helped us to think about helping people to do some of the inviting of others, as well. So, they might invite others over to their own home, out to an event together, or offer a ride to a community meeting.

Some things on the list involve learning, doing something new or exploring. When we try to include these things in a person's day, we find ourselves looking for ways to bring the world to the individual in unique ways. When Brenda was doing some water testing at her park site, one creative Supporter did some dyed water and celery experiments with her to show her the effects of water pollution in her park.

Having the chance to direct something everyday has been a wonderful reminder for us to consider what this means for Tiffany or for Rob who need a focused attempt in order for others to understand their direction. People who care for Tiffany have found ways for her to choose music cassettes and CDs, to turn her own lights on and off, and to open her own front door. One of Rob's Supporters came to understand that Rob was choosing the foods that he wished to buy and eat when he would subtly and silently point at foods in the grocery store. This would have been an easy signal to ignore, but it was not only noticed but even encouraged and strengthened.

Paying attention to all of these items is a way of family, Supporters and others paying a deep respect to the person with a disability. It is a way of providing support among equals.

Role of the Coordinator

We are still learning the importance of maintaining control of our own visions and dreams, and not passing them off to paid Supporters or coordinators. We believe that remembering the importance of this idea will be vital to ensuring a good life for our family members within community.

> *Our way is where family and circle members always maintain control over decision-making, planning, and the routines of daily life. This is the best way that we know of to ensure that our family member remains embedded in real relationships in the community, and does not become a part of the service world which cannot ever replace community. The role of the coordinator and of Supporters is to support, uphold, contribute to, and implement the family vision.*

How We Tell Our Stories: Principles in Action

Telling our stories is our way of inviting others in to think about community and living together in new and wonderful ways.

Early on in our coming together we decided that the best way for us to safeguard the quality of our thinking and the kind of focus that would be expected from us over time would be to limit the size of our group. Although we decided it was better, for a number of reasons, to incorporate and seek charitable status, we consider ourselves to be a family group with a deep history together. We are not a typical 'organization' which seeks to grow and expand in numbers as an indication of the success of our ideas or programs. Therefore, we do not keep a waiting list, we do not engage in membership drives to increase our general membership, and we do not seek out other like-minded people to replicate our 'model' in other places. We are mostly about us and learning how to do things well for ourselves. That, in itself, is hard enough!

However, we are all very much aware of and involved in the lives of many families or individuals without families who are similar to ourselves. So, at the same time that we decided to remain small and focused, we decided that we would take on the role of story teller for other families and individuals who might want to hear about what we had done, were doing, and were learning.

In this light, we meet with families far and wide (many of them come to us to see for themselves) to tell our story. We also tell our story to funders and potential funders, to new and old circle members, to new and old paid Supporters who join us over time, and to our co-operative neighbours and other friends. We find that we need to tell our story to housing officials who make policy, to local politicians who enact by-laws, to community organizations and associations, and to other groups in our community.

Sometimes we tell our big story—the one of our history and how we came to be. Often we begin or focus on our small individual stories with their unique power to impress a clear image. Often we tell our story orally and personally. Sometimes we add overheads and slides to help make our main points. Sometimes, we meet over tea and talk informally with smaller groups. Occasionally, we have had the opportunity to have our story documented by the media through written articles or television documentaries. A few times we have taken the opportunity to write parts of our story on our own. Our book, *We Come Bearing Gifts*, is one such effort, but Linda Dawe and Helen Dionne in particular have written with skill and grace parts of the story too. Some of the Deohaeko families have put together extensive binders that help others come to understand the story of their son or daughter. Some of the families have written vision statements about the kinds of lives their son or daughter wishes to have.

All of these formats—both formal and informal—put our story out in public in some way for others to hear and learn from. In some ways, we are leading very visible lives and we are aware of the responsibility that this holds.

Over time we have come to understand that there are some important components to keep in mind in order to do this part of our work well.

First, with families, it is important to listen to the other families as well as to tell our story. We listen to find out more about the particular path on which another family or finds itself. We listen to find out what part of our story might make the most sense to them. We listen to find out what parts of our story are similar and thus will resonate with them. We listen to allow them to find their own way along the path they are travelling. We have come to understand that we are honoured to have so many families and individuals share with us the unique, joyous and sometimes painful story of their own journey.

Second, we have to allow our stories to come from a deep place. How we tell our story is important. Almost every word placed and every image drawn for others has the ability to uphold or to deny the truth of our whole story. Our stories need to be genuine. They need to be truthful. They need to model the very things that we believe in and stand for.

Third, we need to keep in mind that typical society has a strong stereotype in mind when people think about folks who have a developmental disability. This stereotype often includes images of slowness, unproductive, burden, menace, pity, waste, illness, and ugliness. All of our stories need to counter this negative and false stereotype with positive imagery and stories that depict the more accurate picture of the joy and meaning that these family members bring to our lives. To do this, we try to talk in the following ways:

- Focus on name, age and positive personality characteristics first (musical, good sense of humour, active, gifts).

- Move on to abilities, contributions, possibilities, and dreams—you might have to work on this or enlist others' help, but everyone has some of each of these, only we are not accustomed to thinking and talking in these terms.

- Speak about impairments in every day terms that do not intimidate but give information ("she does not speak" rather than "non-verbal"). Note important limitations and the challenges that these provide "She cannot speak and so we have to make sure that she has other ways to tell us what she needs". Use labels only well into your story and then only when this is helpful to the story and saves a lot of related details—be sure that you have described the person as a unique individual first. Do not deny the impairment, but rather use it to describe the amount and type of support that will be required to live a good life.

- Speak about struggle (if it is appropriate to your story and the audience fits) but make sure that the story is not the struggle. Talk about challenges, fears and struggles within a positive framework. Talk about overcoming the struggle, or about strategies gained and lessons learned.

- End your story with a focus on typical positive roles that the person holds and any achievements they have made within those roles "She has been park steward for 4 years and just received a volunteer award from the city". The best way to ensure that you are doing this is to liken this person's life, hopes, and dreams to those of a peer of the same age in your community who lives a good life and does not have a disability.

Linda Dawe is one of our most prolific speakers and in great demand among family groups across the country. One of the things that make her presentations so memorable and enjoyable is her warm introduction of her daughter, Tiffany.

> Now I'm going to show you some slides about the most important person there is—in my opinion—and that is my daughter Tiffany. Tiffany is a lovely woman who lives her life with courage, dignity, and graciousness. She does many things in typical ways, but getting there is rarely easy. Tiffany is a teacher and contributes much to the lives of people around her.

Most of us end up telling our stories in less grand, but no less important ways. We are telling our story every time we put up a notice in order to find a new Supporter, every time we write a funding proposal or fill out another funding request form, and every time we show and talk about family photographs or show slides that include our family member. We tell our stories during every orientation with a new Supporter, and in every piece of paper that we use to track the various things that we think need to be tracked in writing about our family member. We tell our stories in circle meetings, in related gatherings with other members, in hallways and lobbies with friends and neighbours, and with colleagues who know little about our lives. Let's look into these other ways a bit more closely.

When we write a job posting and we want to attract energetic, creative people who can make some kind of a commitment, we would do well to follow the pointers listed above. We need to think about writing a job posting as building an invitation. We need to begin the invitation with words that tell of at least four positive qualities of the individual. These can include characteristics or personal qualities, personal interests (especially if they are impressive, familiar, and age-appropriate), special skills or activities, and gifts. Our posting must demonstrate the basic respect and values that will characterize the rest of their experience within our family.

We need to talk about our loved ones—tell their stories and our stories, so to speak—in rich, full ways that will attract people who want to make a difference. If that rich, full life is not yet happening, we need to describe the kinds of dreams and visions that we and our family members might hold for the future. The posting of such a notice is a public event. Everyone who reads it gets a piece of the story. Even if they do not know us, or do not meet us in this process, we are contributing to their understanding of the situation of people with disabilities in their community. Let's make a positive contribution to that story. Here is one example of an effort to write a job posting that tells a small part of a fuller story:

> *A woman in her thirties, who has been named as the environmental steward of a park site along Frenchman's Bay, is looking for an enthusiastic, creative assistant to help her pursue her environmental interests and duties. She attends her sites daily to perform a variety of upkeep, observation, and data collection tasks. Hands-on gardening, collecting, recording, and nature craft projects would all be of interest for this woman's time on site or back at home.*

Orientation sessions with new Supporters, or just getting to know a new neighbour or circle member better are further opportunities when we cannot help but tell our story. Once again, when we use the above steps or points to give us direction, we can tell a positive story with many places for new Supporters or others to find a place to give of their own skills and talents.

Sometimes, we use photo albums or even slides to give people a visual sense of our family member in terms of their roles, activities, and relationships. These are very powerful ways to tell a story. However, we find that taking the most positively powerful photograph needs to be a conscious act of an aware person. We must be aware of the subtle messages that our photos might be showing. It is easy to show many photos of a person going about their business, but without one other person in the picture. We have found that photographs give complementary and strong, positive messages about the person when they show people in strong roles or in relationship with others. If the photos are mainly concerned with the person on their own, one may wonder about why no one else is interested in this person. If the photos typically show the other people to be paid support workers, the very same question might arise. If however, we can gather a groups of photos and slides that show a range of family, neighbours, friendly bankers and shopkeepers, a very different message is sent.

In the same way, we can make sure that photos and slides reflect the person actively holding strong, positive roles in their life. When people are seen as working at familiar jobs, partaking in typical leisure pursuits, and joining in well-known sports events a powerful message is sent about the common ground that this person shares with the listener. Even when the challenge for the new Supporter is to help create a week and a life that looks more like that in the future (but does not now), it is possible to make sure that photographs include a smaller, but still positive range of family relations. Also there are low key roles that can be picked up on film. A sports fan can be photographed in his room decorated with all of the paraphernalia. A family member can be seen helping with chores, setting the table, hanging out with siblings, and so on.

We also use all kinds of written material that help us to tell the story of the person. We try to make sure that written documentation happens only for things that need to be tracked, rather than for idle curiosity or less important reasons. These are then tracked in as unobtrusive formats as possible. We also use written forms that can give good information about a person and their life experiences. Several of the people connected with Deohaeko Support Network have a binder of information. Sometimes these are titled, *About Jon* for example, and they are a respectful compilation of good information about Jon, his likes and dislikes, what others say about him and how they know him, a written vision for a path into the future, and lots of other details. These books can contain health information, family stories to fill out the story of the person's whole life, and emergency information as well. We have developed an extensive list of a possible table of contents for such books. The collection of information is based on all of the things that we think the person might want to let another person know as their relationship unfolds.

Funding proposals are another opportunity for us to decide just how we want to tell our story. Oftentimes, families feel compelled to tell their story in ways that emphasize their stress at the lack of funding, or our failures due to lack of resources. We have enjoyed very good success in refusing to speak about our family members and our families in these ways. We try, instead, to tell the stories that illustrate the efforts of a person to live as full a life as possible while experiencing some practical limitations that make some things difficult. We ask for assistance in helping the individual reach their own typical and familiar goals. We emphasize how family, friends, and others have gone out of their way to support the individual as much as possible, and point out further ways that resources are needed to help this along. In the end, our resource request may not be any different than a funding proposal where a family tells of its weakness and burdens, but we feel stronger and renewed in the joy of our family member by this way of sharing our story with potential funders.

Here are a couple of examples of excerpts, written by a mother, from one of our earliest funding proposals.

Brenda is supported to live in her apartment at Rougemount Co-operative with some support dollars and large amounts of my time and support. I am not getting any younger and feel the strain of managing two homes, while at the same time needing to support my own elderly mother. I am thrilled that Brenda has found a place where she truly feels at home. I worry that Brenda's new-found sense of home is at risk because of the over-reliance on my support to make this work. If something should happen to me, she would not have enough support to continue to call Rougemount home. At the same time, due to the attention our community pays to developing and maintaining natural community supports and connections, paid support costs for Brenda will always be lower for her in this environment than in any other setting. This proposal seeks to secure a range of supports to Brenda in her home, so that her future at Rougemount is more assured.

1. Goals and Results

With the additional support dollars, I hope to secure Brenda's place at Rougemount well into the future. We would be able to honour Brenda's choice of Rougemount Co-operative as her home.

Additional support dollars would provide Brenda with some much needed evening support. Especially at times when a roommate is not in place, Brenda finds the evening hours long and lonely. I expect that more evening support would help Brenda to participate more in evening events, to take a more active role in preparing her own evening meal, and to begin to host small gatherings in her home so that she begins to feel more comfortable in reaching out and inviting people in when she is lonely.

Some weekend support would allow Brenda to spend more weekend time in her apartment and in her community instead of at our family home. From our experience, we know that natural supports are strengthened when the person is present during the events in the life of the community. These dollars would increase Brenda's presence and result in stronger and more natural connections within the Rougemount community.

In summary, the extra support dollars proposed would ensure that Brenda spends time in her home, based on her inclination and desires, rather than based on when support is available or I am able to be with her in the co-operative.

We are aware that our actions and decisions in many ways tell our story and demonstrate the nature of our principles in action more clearly than any Principles document. Throughout this book, I will continue to tell many of our stories in the best ways that I can. Each will tell its own story about our principles, but also about our struggles, our transient successes, and our higher hopes for the future. The stories that I tell are always in transition. The ones that I put down on paper have already changed into something new. New stories are being lived this very moment. This represents a challenge to us in having to find renewed energy every day to work on what's new and different. But it also represents our hope in knowing that what is not yet good will certainly change, and our biggest problems today will lie behind by tomorrow.

Let me end with a fuller story to show how our principles in action help us to define and make decisions in our daily life.

Becoming an Artist

Two years ago, Tiffany was dabbling with paint. Now, she is becoming an artist. What has made the difference? Thoughtfulness, clear intent and planning.

Two years ago, Tiffany started to play around with some water colours, in part because one of her Supporters was an artist and had begun to notice Tiffany's interest in colour and beauty around her, and in part because Tiffany sometimes had some spare time on her hands. We were always conscious of looking for home-based hobbies and options that would give Tiffany a further sense of well being and contentment in her own home.

In the beginning, Tiffany painted away fairly privately and quietly. Diane, her Supporter, discovered that Tiffany much preferred to approach her art in very, quiet, intimate surroundings. She seemed to be most focused and attentive to work in the small bedroom, with the door closed, no one else in the apartment and only Diane by her side. In time, Tiffany produced a quantity of private work of a quality that seemed to please them both. At that point, Diane helped her design a few paintings into Christmas and greeting cards.

The reception of these cards was immediate and enthusiastic. Requests for cards, whole paintings and more came swiftly from family, circle members and neighbours.

However, there was a catch. Very early on, it became clear that Tiffany was turning out to be a temperamental painter—someone who could only work when the Muse struck her. Diane believes that this characteristic has saved Tiffany as an artist. Since her production was totally unpredictable, they began to tell people not to expect any cards or paintings for a while to come. That allowed Tiffany the time, space and emotional opportunity to further explore her talent without any pressure to move into high production.

So, Tiffany continued to paint and experiment behind closed doors, with mainly Diane to view her work and understand the importance of this period. This gave Tiffany alone the control over whether or not she wanted to paint. And as she continued to choose to paint, and obviously delight in her own work, she began to choose to be an artist.

When both Tiffany and Diane felt that Tiffany was firmly choosing this direction, they slowly began to show Tiffany's art to the people around her. She made and laser-copied some more cards. She made a few framed water colours as gifts. Tiffany framed three of her paintings to hang in her own living room and began to enjoy the comments of neighbours and guests in her home.

Over time, Diane helped Tiffany to save some of her paintings and begin to have a 'body of work'—an identifiable style and approach that was hers alone. Tiffany joined a local Art Centre, and as a member went often to view other member's art, volunteer with other member artists at lawn parties and other guild functions, and generally explore the life of an art guild member. Twice she displayed her art at the members' art show.

After discussion with her circle members, Tiffany decided to enter one of her watercolours into a juried art show put on by the Pine Ridge Art Council in Ajax. In a juried show, work is judged before it is accepted into the show. Tiffany's art was not chosen for that show, but she was not deterred from painting, since many other artists were juried out as well. Tiffany has shown her art on other occasions involving small home shows with fellow Durham Region artists. Although sales have been small, Tiffany's art has been well received.

At one point, Tiffany's mother received a request for Tiffany to show her art at the end of a one-day conference. After much thought and discussion among those of us closest to Tiffany and her art, this offer was declined. The reasons for this were varied and important. In the first place, Tiffany had not yet had an official exhibit of her own work, and probably, as an artist, was not quite ready for one. Secondly, we wanted this occasion when it happened, to take place in a truly wonderful venue, as only fitting for a first exhibit. This particular venue was fine, but not lovely or particularly focused on her art. Thirdly, the conference in question was one that would draw people together who were interested in issues of disability. We thought that Tiffany's fledgling identity as an artist would be overshadowed by her identity as a woman with a disability in such an environment. Once again, we wanted to make sure that Tiffany's opportunities in her role of artist would be separate and distinct from any deliberate focus on her disability. In order to do this, she needed to be seen mostly among typical artists, and mostly among art-loving people who would come to her event because of their love of art, not mainly to support a good cause.

Today, Tiffany continues to paint, and struggles to find the funds to frame her artwork and for show entry fees. Like many artists, she continues to search for ways to show her art to the public, beyond the loving reach of family and close friends. Some of her paintings and cards are on display for sale at a local shop. She also continues to keep her eye open for the right venue for her 'opening' show. When the time is right, and circumstances are ready, Tiffany will exhibit her art.

Section 2
A Growing Sense of Belonging

Chapter 3: Home is the First Place
Chapter 4: Tending to Relationship
Chapter 5: A Greater Sense of Place

What does it mean to be rooted in community? It means that there are places where you are recognized, helped, encouraged and welcomed into playing important roles. It means that you experience this belonging in a number of different spaces—your own home, your co-operative, your neighbourhood shopping places, your place of work, local civic places, your places of leisure, and your social gathering places including others' homes. Each space represents another root system so that several together represent a life better situated in community than a life with only one root.

Being rooted in community means that you are of the people. You encounter daily a wide variety of people to meet you, to greet you, miss you when you are not there, welcome your contributions, enjoy your presence and support your participation. And in your turn, you meet them, greet them, miss them, appreciate their contributions, and enjoy their presence. Some of those people will also come into your home and your life more intimately and personally and come be with you in committed ways. Their presence will make a difference in your life and you in theirs. These relationships which become personal and committed represent a full, deep root system. The others are various root hairs and offshoots, still vital and important to sustain life in your community.

Being rooted in community means that you have several valued, well-recognized roles that you play within your community. These roles give you places to be, people to be with, contributions to make, activities to undertake, responsibilities to manage, and a presence in community. These include major identifying roles (mother, daughter, sister, brother), civic roles (co-operative member, campaign worker, voting citizen), work roles (gardener, teacher's helper, burger flipper, dishwasher, environmental steward, small business owner, baker, artist), leisure roles (social activist, guild member, bird watcher, team coach), and relationship roles (friend, confidante, listener). Each role places another root burrowing down into the earth.

Being well rooted in your community means that people do not talk about you "going out into the community for the day". You are in community where you are. Community has come to you. You are of the community. You live and breathe in the community. You cannot pull yourself out of it at night only to re-enter at will the next day. You spend time in a home of your own choosing, into which you invite a variety of family, friends, and others. This is community. You live as a full member in a housing co-operative where you put in your helping hours, vote in elections, participate in decision-making processes and take good care of your neighbours. This is community. You make significant contributions to the economic life of your community with your many volunteer hours, your local shopping, and your use of local services. This is community. Being rooted in community means belonging.

Being rooted in community is all about belonging—the eternal human quest that gives life meaning and value. We have come to see that in some situations belonging does not just happen. In our society which generally values speed over slowness, productivity over presence, standardized and prescribed beauty over unique beauty, uniformity over variety, and elitism over tolerance and inclusion, belonging does not happen spontaneously or easily for many members who fall outside the mould. The sons and daughters of Deohaeko families are some such members of society. For them, as for all vulnerable people at the margins of society, belonging must be studied and understood, and consciously planned and developed. The pathway to belonging needs to be rebuilt, even somewhat contrived, so that these members might have access to the same opportunities.

The foundation of this pathway has already been set. We have articulated a firm set of values and principles. We are rooted in typical community life, many of us within an intentional community experience. We have gathered together a group of good, thoughtful people. Now, in this next section, we turn our attention to three solid elements that will guide and support people forward into the opportunities that life can afford them.

Home is the first sense of place, representing security and identity. A warm, solid home base where the person experiences much control will become the stronghold from which people may venture to experience other parts of life.

Belonging means being **in relationship** with one another. Our experiences with circles of support and larger supportive networks are vital to the context of relationship and belonging. They are the key to ensuring positive futures for our sons and daughters because they are a way of focusing on relationship for and with the person. The forces of society that do not value the lives and presence of our sons and daughters are such that we must surround them with a group of protective and safe-guarding souls who will work together to provide the opportunities to the person. People need to have many places to be, roles to hold and people to be with. This takes the time, energy, synergy and enthusiasm of a group of people. Furthermore, the outcomes and celebrations deserve to be shared by a small crowd, at least.

Finally, our experiences in **community spaces** outside of our homes have been a wide learning experience for all of us. We will share our thoughts and experiences of the kinds of community spaces to which our family members might belong, and the kind of community spaces in which we all may thrive. This is clearly the point at which healthy spaces in community for our family members who are vulnerable, are also healthy spaces for us all.

Our understanding of becoming rooted in community is about figuring out belonging—a place to call home, good relationships, and good places to welcome us away from home. The stories in the three chapters of this section are stories about finding and defining one's home, about reaching out in relationship, and about discovering good community spaces. These stories show us that the ideas in these chapters are not just abstract ideas, but rather the truth of experience that we have learned by following and sharing in the lives of Brenda, Caroline, Donna, John, Jon, Rob and Tiffany.

Chapter 3
Home is the First Place

Home is the first sense of place. Our early work sought to truly involve our sons and daughters in the building of the co-operative, in choosing their own apartment units, in buying furniture, painting and decorating, and finally in becoming as involved as possible in choosing roommates, Supporters, and others who might come into their homes. This began to pay off as the sense of ownership was felt by each person. There was—and is—a general sense of ease and security in one's home and the feeling that each person's place was truly home to them. Thus, each person's first sense of place outside of the family home became a positive and concrete experience.

Looking back we can see this link between a firm sense of home and a greater sense of identity developing. People were growing and maturing in their sense of self and identity. People were feeling good about the safety and security they felt within their homes and used this as a foundation to develop a fuller identity. People were doing just the kind of exploring, experimenting and learning that we had wished and hoped for and in their exploring they were coming to some conclusions about their spaces and places, their tastes and yearnings. This was not always clear to us at the time. Sometimes, it was hard to see the forest for the trees and what it felt like was a series of dilemmas and situations that were not easy to sort out.

We learned many things about people's sense of home and many of these can be summed up by noting a series of images that have greeted us at various moments over the past eight years. These images generated questions and discussions among ourselves. This was clearly a time of learning for us all.

Whose Home is It?

Image: Dropping in to see Rob while a Supporter is there with him, and the lovely Slovakian couple who share his apartment spend some quiet time in their tiny bedroom. Why is everyone whispering?

Image: Every time I stop by Rob's place that he now shares with a new roommate, I see another piece of furniture or another picture that was not there before. Slowly we realize that this feels less and less like Rob's place and more like Rob living in someone else's home.

Image: There is a stranger sleeping on Brenda's couch when she wakes up one Saturday morning. She does not like it and feels very upset. Who is she? It turns out that Brenda's new roommate took pity on a stranger at a local fair who had no place to sleep. This met the roommate's sense of home, but what did it do for Brenda's?

Image: Tiffany and family decide to forego the supportive roommate model, and simply advertise for a room for rent. Sandy wants a room and access to a kitchen and bathroom. She works long hours with a family in the area and she has many relatives where she wants to be on the weekends. All she really wants is a small, congenial space for herself. She stays as Tiffany's roommate for over five years.

Image: John lived with a roommate for a year and then determinedly struck out on his own. When you enter his apartment now, you quickly get a full and accurate account of John's interests and passions. Toronto Maple Leaf paraphernalia cover the walls, and line the shelves. Game schedules and statistics cover a corner of his sofa. A computer sits in one corner surrounded by family photos. A large video collection fills one bookcase. Although John is a shy man, it is easy to draw him into conversation about the passions that so obviously fill his life.

The images above lead us to the question: *Whose home is it?* This is how we began to answer this question.

Through Rob's various experiences, we came to understand that we must ensure that this is Rob's home. Rob is the priority for us. Rob is the one who will not likely be able to experience and create his own sense of home without our thoughtfulness and support.

If it is Rob's home, it should look like Rob and feel like Rob, and tell us something about Rob. Rob's interest in music, his love of horses, and his preference for an uncluttered apartment lay out are subtle and newly emerging aspects of Rob's sense of home. However, when he shares his home with someone else, he begins to lose his sense of home. Even very caring and sensitive roommates cannot help but overwhelm Rob with their presence. The small aspects of Rob's personality and interests begin to disappear. Roommates of Rob's age have acquired a significant amount of 'stuff', including a wealth of experience to help them design a home that they desire. Favourite chairs and pictures, ways of organizing the kitchen, foods and smells, all quickly identify their presence and mask Rob's. A roommate cannot help but take over the sense of home by sheer weight of his own experiences compared to Rob's over the same period of time. The typical roommate has more stuff, more determined tastes and preferences, more friends, and more freedom to come and go. He knows what it takes with a few quick moves to make the apartment feel like home to him. In doing so, some of Rob's fragile presence is erased.

When we first started helping Rob look for a roommate, we thought we were looking for someone to enter into a life sharing experience. With Rob's various experiences (living alone, living with one roommate, living with a couple, living alone but with more space) we came to better understand just what we were looking for. We saw that having a roommate is not the same as having a life sharing opportunity, nor is it the same as having someone simply sleep over in your home to ensure your well-being. Life sharing involves a commitment over the very long term, and would allow for a slow process of moving in and growing together in ways that would not overwhelm the individual's identity. In life sharing there is a whole life ahead to create space. We did not feel that we were at a point of even wanting this degree of life sharing and we realized that our search for a roommate was a different matter altogether.

With a roommate you are involved with another individual who wants their own sense of home right away (or soon) so that they can get on with their own life. Ironically, the greater sense of home that the roommate feels, the longer they will likely stay. However, the greater sense of home is almost always made, albeit unintentionally, at the expense of Rob or Jon or Brenda's sense of home.

Rob is in the early stages of figuring out who he is and what he prefers in his home. This sense of identity is still very fragile and easily overtaken. Rob's home can be so quickly made to feel like someone else's place. He may be content there, but it will not be a refuge for him. It will not be the sense of place and belonging that launches him confidently for some of that same sense of belonging into other community spaces. At this time Rob most wants and needs an opportunity to define his own home on his own terms. This will take time, space, and opportunity. A support person—who does not want or need to call this home—sleeping over in a second bedroom can best afford him these conditions.

On the other hand, John's home demonstrates to us what happens when a person is able to fully grow into and define for himself, a place called 'home'. It is comfortable to John, and he is proud to talk about these aspects of his life. It gives others clear messages about areas of common interest and emphasizes the ways in which John is similar to others of his age, and yet uniquely himself.

Brenda's experience with her surprise visitor told us that her roommate did not understand Brenda's extreme vulnerability, or her intense need to feel her home as a secure and inviolable place where surprises and uncertainties would be few. The roommate so quickly felt her own sense of home within Brenda's apartment that she felt free to offer it to someone else. She denied Brenda the sense of home, by asserting her own feelings first. She forgot to allow Brenda a part in the decision, and in doing so robbed Brenda of one of the primary characteristics of home—personal security.

Tiffany's situation is different. It is important to understand some of the reasons that having a typical roommate work for her. For one thing, she advertised for a room for rent and initially gave exactly that—an attractive room with no other expectations. The friendship and caring that grew over the years was given ample opportunity to flourish due to the things that we know can work—presence, time, mutual attraction, shared interests and shared spaces. However, in the beginning Tiffany was simply offering what Sandy wanted and needed—a small space of her own. Another important factor was one of space. Tiffany lives in a spacious three bedroom apartment with two bathrooms. There was space enough to accommodate Tiffany, a family member, a Supporter and a visitor without crowding. Thirdly, an important factor was that Sandy did not want to recreate her full home life within Tiffany's apartment. She had family elsewhere and happily travelled to be with them on weekends. Her home life with Tiffany was small and contained. So, in essence, Tiffany managed to find a person who never questioned or challenged whose home it was. Over time, Sandy also came to understand how important it was for Tiffany to maintain a solid identity as the primary owner of that home.

These images and ensuing discussions helped us to understand the importance of home for each of the sons and daughters of the families. We became firmly convinced that we needed to assist people to establish their own sense of home, and while we might have empathy for the plights of roommates also searching for home our energy needed to focus on our own family members first. This would always be an area of extreme vulnerability for each of them. A strong home centre would provide a safe haven, a springboard, and a place of welcome—all links to other parts of their lives. This would be some of the strongest roots that they would set down within their new lives.

Here is another set of images and questions:

When It is Too Crowded, Who Leaves?

Image: I am talking with Mary, Jon's mother, about Jon's circle in Jon's tiny dining room area. Jon is in the living room just an arm's length away looking at a home video in which he stars. Pat, a Supporter, is in the kitchen baking up another cake to bring to tonight's Rosary Group potluck in the co-operative. Out of the second bedroom comes roommate Jason, followed by his girlfriend, on their way out for dinner. It is crowded, busy and noisy in Jon's home.

Image: a couple of times when Brenda was upset in her apartment, she threw her purse on the ground, yelled at the Supporter, grabbed her keys and ran out into the hallway and out the front door. This caused a great deal of worry for her safety while outside, distraught and near to local traffic. We also realize that in her distress Brenda is turning away from home, rather than moving toward it. Something is wrong.

Image: Rob's sharing arrangement has fallen through and to avoid being moved for being 'over housed', he is helped to move to a one bedroom unit with a Supporter who sleeps over. On the many restless nights when Rob needs to pace in the darkness while sleep eludes him, he stumbles over the Supporter's pull-out couch bed. Rob is anxious and confused. What has happened to his living room? Why can't he roam around like he always does? During the daytime, Mom and Dad drop by with some supplies and go to arrange them in his bedroom. Someone drops in for tea. The Supporter is in the kitchen. Rob is overwhelmed by the number of people and the amount of activity in his apartment. He can only escape into his bedroom and his parents leave to give him some quiet.

Image: Rob and Jon both move to two-bedroom apartments where they live without roommates, and have someone sleep over in the second bedrooms. They feel a greater sense of space and refuge in their own home. There is more space for the number of people who come and go in their lives. When things start to feel crowded, all of the people have another place to go (the second bedroom). Regional housing puts out a message that they feel this may be 'over housing'. An overnight support person does not qualify as a roommate for the purposes of providing housing (support persons already have their own home). People may need to move to one-bedroom units, or return to the roommate model. Brenda has lived in her unit for 8 years, most of that time without a roommate, and feels it is the most stable and secure place in her life. Rob has tried a one-bedroom unit and we know it does not work for him. Jon feels crowded enough in his two-bedroom unit, without returning to the roommate option.

The question that comes to discussion is: *When it is too crowded, who leaves?*

When Jon's home is full and too crowded, who gets pushed out? There was no easy answer to this question at first. Jon's Mom needs to be present spontaneously and freely to keep her finger on the pulse of the atmosphere in Jon's home. She must be welcomed at all times. The roommate is a person without another home. He needs to feel somewhat free to find space and use the common areas in the apartment. When it is crowded, where does he go? How long will he stay under these circumstances? How will that instability affect Jon? How do we meet the reasonable needs of a roommate without it being at the cost of Jon's sense of home? Shall Jon be asked to leave his own home, or the Supporter? Neither of these makes sense if the overall goal is to help Jon experience and create a refuge of belonging and control and call it home.

We have come to more fully understand the value of space for Jon and others. In Jon's crowded situation, it was decided that he should try to live without a roommate. A sleepover Supporter began to spend the night at Jon's in his second bedroom. A few things happened. For one, we realized that in part due to the sheer number of bodies around, Jon and his roommate actually had not spend much quality time together—one of the main reasons for choosing a roommate model in the first place. We think that the roommate was out a lot because the apartment felt full, but we also could not find natural ways for Jon and his roommate to spend much time together. Another advantage without the roommate was that now there was a second bedroom to retire into when things got busy. Previously, it was the roommate's private space and could not be used. Now it was Jon's second bedroom, used for a variety of purposes but empty during the day. Mary could go there to make a phone call or talk with someone quietly. The Supporter could go in there and give Jon a sense of privacy and space within his living quarters.

It became clear to us why a one-bedroom apartment would not work for Jon. Jon is reliant on other people for his support at all times. This means that there is *always* a second person (usually unrelated) in his apartment. That is the general criterion of adequate housing—you are afforded a two bedroom apartment when two people (deemed not a couple) live in the same apartment. The only catch is that in Jon's case the second person already has their own home. But from his living point of view, there is always a second person in his home. Authorities may not agree with us in the end, but we are clearer on the value of space and what works for Jon. This has worked out in similar ways for both Rob and Brenda. There is space for a person to spend the night, but not for a person to move in and remove a bedroom from general accessibility.

When it is too crowded, we need to focus on the vulnerable person first. The individual person and the one person (family, paid support, friend) needed to make sure they are well is the basic unit. We place this first, and design other supports and interactions as it works for the person. For Rob, Brenda, and Jon the roommate option provided too much crowding without enough opportunity for compensatory relationship. Once again, we are reminded of the vulnerability of the people we care about. We must put them first.

The soundness of this strategy has been underlined by Brenda's reaction to being upset in her own home. With a focus on Brenda, it was pretty easy to figure out what to do. It's Brenda's home and when she is upset, *we* leave, not her. Her reaction to our leaving has shown us that this works for her. Even when Brenda runs out first, we have discovered that if the Supporter quickly and visibly leaves and goes to sit in the lobby Brenda quickly returns to her home. Her home is her castle. It's her place to be upset. It ought to be her refuge and her security. We are only present at her welcome.

The next series of images include:

A Place of Home or a Place of Work?

Image: I walk into Brenda's home. There is a support schedule hanging on her fridge. An enthusiastic student has posted a personal hygiene chart on her bathroom wall. As I go into the second bedroom where Brenda allows me to keep a phone and a desk (there is also a bed, a closetful of Brenda's off-season clothing, and a collection of art supplies), a Supporter says there is a note for me "in the office".

Image: I am sitting with Tiffany in her living room listening to a new CD, and aware of a new Supporter in her kitchen, talking on her cell phone to a friend who called to make plans for after work. The Supporter is young, fashionable and sporting short cut-off shorts and a t-shirt that does not cover her midriff. She's decided that she should wear casual clothing such as she wears at home in this new home-centred job.

These images, and a hundred like them, brought us to many discussions about: *Is this a place of home or a place of work?*

We have learned that there is a fundamental conflict when we pay someone to assist a person in their home to make a home. It is a home for the person with a disability. It is a place of work for the Supporter. We must acknowledge this essential conflict, and understand how we work with it will have great impact on Brenda's or Tiffany's sense of home. The Supporter needs to be helped to understand the priority of their support is to help the individual create their own sense of home.

Jo Masserelli of the *SRV Implementation Project* in Massachusetts and Joe Osburn from the *Indiana Safeguards Initiative* have put a lot of thought into this fundamental conflict between work space and home life. In a one-day workshop entitled *Strangers in the House* they explore the dilemma of preserving home and home life while receiving much-needed in-home supports. They start off with the premise that reflects our experience succinctly: when families or individuals need extra help and rely on paid support coming into the home there is *always* a dilemma because it necessarily intrudes on home and family life. There is a clash between the need for help and the need for a private family life.

In some ways, simply acknowledging this fundamental conflict has been very helpful to us. We know it to be true. Supporters leave home and arrive with parameters, expectations and goals for their work day that can make the supported person feel like they are not 'at home' within their home. Things that make the Supporter's work easier (charts, schedules, communication books, open conversations about intimate details) can quickly make a home feel like someone's place of work. At the same time, the casual nature of the setting, and often the casual ways that we go about finding and hiring Supporters, lead them to assume that there are fewer rules and lower expectations than in other work settings. That is when we see extremely casual dress and personal telephone calls at all hours.

Once we realized this basic conflict between support and typical private life, we felt free to make changes and exert positive influence where we could.

We have found that acknowledging the conflict up front to new Supporters is very helpful. "This is a work setting for you, but it is a home for Brenda." We ask that they respect this conflict and do their utmost to minimize it. I find it useful for them to ask themselves whether they would take similar actions in their own homes. Would they put a list in the bathroom about what personal hygiene routines are expected each morning? Would they (or their spouse) talk to casual neighbours about their bathroom habits, cycles or moods?

We talk to Supporters about making the paperwork as natural and contained as possible. Many people have a small home office in their living space. This is appropriate and familiar, but the contents are usually kept private and in their place. We ask them to be aware of and remove any unnecessary signs to neighbours and friends that this is a place of work, rather than Brenda's apartment. In this way health and medication records can be kept in a drawer and taken out only when in use. A drawer in a small home desk can be designated for schedules, invoices, pay cheques, etc. Schedules and plans work best on a typical calendar that shares the information, again from the individual's point of view. When this is attractively done, with a focus on roles and activities it also serves as point of communication for visitors to one's home. It is also helpful when work schedules are kept out of sight, or written unobtrusively on calendars.

Sometimes written communication is desirable, and so we try to encourage ways for it to happen in an anecdotal form (in the first person). In that way when it is read back it provides an interesting account of the person's day, much like a personal journal, e.g., "and after supper, we quickly did dishes because we wanted to get over to Marje's and deliver the fruit salad we had made for her. She was delighted with it and asked us to stay for a cup of tea". This is also an excellent way to ensure that people are written about in positive and supportive ways. In several situations, these journals are brought to other family members on weekends and used as a way of the person sharing a bit about their week. Reading a well-written journal together has been a loving and bonding experience. Attentive Supporters have contributed to this well.

It is often helpful to have a conversation about the use of cell phones these days. Before general cell phone use, it was rare for Supporters to receive personal phone calls during their support hours. The few calls that were received were generally genuine family emergencies and families were happy to provide the telephone link to help the situation. Today, almost every Supporter carries a cell phone, often with clear advantages to the health and safety of the individual. At the same time, we have noticed that the number of phone calls both to and from the Supporter's family and friends has escalated. When the Supporter is on paid time, both the work and the home environments are being violated. This is a place of work for the Supporter and the majority of the phone calls are inappropriate and a waste of the individual's time and support dollars. At the same time, the personal calls for a Supporter into the individual's home violate the individual's sense of home. They are an intrusion into his private domain, they waste his personal time, and they bring discussions into his home which have nothing to do with him or his time. He is ignored and rendered invisible—while paying for the time!

It is also helpful to talk with paid Supporters about which parts of their job are really like a typical work role. There are often subtle, but important, expectations around punctuality, reliability, appropriate and enhancing dress, communication, health and safety. Things work best when these potentially cloudy areas are clarified when the person first starts.

Place of home. Place of work. Yes, there is an essential conflict, but one that can be used as a point for learning greater respect and appreciation of the challenge of the task for us to help people gain a sense of home.

These experiences and questions were all brought to us by the people who receive support or by those that care about them deeply. They were saying, by their actions, moods and words, that their home had become important to them and that when it wasn't working for them something had to be done. It is not always easy to listen well. We are not always able to make the right decisions right away.

Rob has tried out several living arrangements. Although it has certainly caused him some difficulty, he has also become clearer with us on what he wants from a home. He communicates this to us in many ways, and we collect those bits of information and put them together, making changes and moves as the opportunities become available to us.

Rob is in a very dynamic process of defining home for himself. We do not think that it is a coincidence that at the same time as we have been able to make accommodations to better suit his definition of home, Rob has been active and involved about seeking out other community spaces of welcome.

Rob's experience with home has been an essentially satisfying one, perhaps giving him the confidence or the taste for trying out some more. Home is the first community space where Rob has felt the glow of belonging and welcome. We believe that from there, he has gone out to search (and find) more spaces where some of the same elements of welcome and belonging exist.

Caroline Ann also taught us a lot when she began to define home for herself. We had a vague idea when we started out that we were making an important and life-defining decisions on behalf of and with our children that home would be Rougemount Co-operative. We also said that this was the current place people would call home and this might change over time. And all of this came to pass. Caroline Ann is the first person who has helped us take the leap away from defining home as 'home in Rougemount'.

Caroline Ann talked, dreamed and described home to her family and circle members often over seven years. At some point, circle members—and especially her mother, Helen—realized that her Rougemount apartment, so lovingly decorated with Toronto Maple Leaf blue and Scottish tartan, would never match the dream in her head. Caroline Ann has experienced and enjoyed Rougemount and come to understand that she has the key role in defining her home. And it's in a different place altogether.

Caroline Ann was able to articulate and appreciate the many benefits and relationships she had come to enjoy at Rougemount. She had friends, people to get together with during the day, and neighbours to look out for her when she was in need (during thunder storms, or when she ran out of garbage bags). As office kitchen organizer, members' meeting coffee server, and office helper she made a contribution to the co-operative that was valuable and welcomed. She lived across the street from a Montessori school where she volunteered regularly. Having lived the experience of the co-operative apartment building life, she began to make comparisons and evaluations. In the end, she was able to articulate what would mean home to her.

As we listened to her over many months, it was clear that the image of home for Caroline Ann was synonymous with a residential, suburban neighbourhood with single family dwellings. For her, home would be a house where one went outside to take out the garbage and shovel snow, and had direct access to gardens. Home would be a neighbourhood where one walked along streets where one could be seen and called to from nearby homes. Home would be a place where she had much better access to her family—especially her young nephew, Terry—when she wanted it, rather than waiting for rides to be arranged.

At first we tried in many ways to see if we could make Rougemount work for her. We talked about moving to a first floor apartment with access to the ravine. We talked about her taking on roles with snow shovelling and garbage collection. But Caroline Ann's perseverance taught us to listen. Caroline Ann's circle slowly came to the realization that Rougemount did not and could not fit the ideal picture of 'home' in Caroline Ann's mind. Even as we worried that we would not be able to find just what she wanted, we promised to try and investigate and see what we could do. She was very patient with us. Our search of alternatives took over two years. We really learned a lot about listening and not limiting dreams.

Over the months, we investigated apartments in the family neighbourhood where she had lived with her family for many years. These were expensive and tended to be poorly-lit basement apartments which her family could not bring themselves to appreciate. In the end, Helen and George felt the right thing to do was to renovate their home, and build a separate apartment for their daughter. Being the high profile president of Deohaeko Support Network, renown for her part building the Rougemount Co-operative, and helping so many families in her community work, this could not have been an easy decision for Helen. On the face of it, others might well judge this decision as taking a step back. However, Helen and George demonstrated their commitment to listening to their daughter, not just when they thought they knew the answer, but also when the answer was hard to hear.

Helen's courage to listen and walk with her daughter is a significant model to many families who also know the right thing to do in their hearts even when it runs against the tide. As it is, the true answer to the question, "Why has she moved? Didn't it work out?" is that, "Yes, actually it did work out". And like with many things done rightly, it has worked out for many reasons and in many ways. Caroline Ann found out that she will be listened to by people who know and love her well. Her circle has learned a powerful lesson about listening to Caroline Ann. She has grown in her ability to describe what she wants and needs in her life. She is happy with her new home, with her neighbourhood, and with her contact with her family. In many ways, Caroline Ann may not have been able to figure out her sense of home without the seven years in the co-operative.

As for Caroline Ann, she has returned to volunteer at the local elementary school in her neighbourhood. She meets and greets neighbours outside all of the time. She maintains her ties with Rougemount and finds ways to get over every week or so. She is learning how to make those visits coincide with her friends being free to see her. She has discovered that her sister comes over to her parent's home more often since the arrival of their son a couple of years ago, and so her role of 'aunt' and 'sister' are developing in wonderful and natural ways. Before, there was always the juggle of how she would get a ride in order to 'pop in' at her parent's when her sister was there. Now she's just naturally there.

This is a fairly recent story about home, but it is one that has helped me to realize that it is not only Caroline, but all of the others as well, who have been deeply involved with defining 'home' for themselves. As people have struggled with roommates, the size of their units, décor, deciding on what happens within their homes and more, they have been involved with telling us how they want to define home in very personal terms.

Currently, home for Rob is a spacious two-bedroom apartment where he can roam day and night without encountering pull-out couches or crowded rooms. It is the place where his long sofa awaits him on days when he is not feeling well. It is also the place where he only has to get up and stand before the door in order for a sensitive Supporter or family member to accompany him into the other welcoming spaces in his community.

For Jon, home is the place where he can safely display his enthusiastic seasonal decorations without overwhelming others and for as long as he wishes. It is a place where he exerts a lot of control over what to do and when to do it.

John has defined a home for himself as shown above, a home which accommodates him and his interests in fully satisfying ways. Donna's home is a place of family. It is where she and Matthew spend much of their time, and it is where Donna has positioned the china cabinet she inherited from her mother. A large poster of Marje adorns her hallway, and many photos line her bookshelves.

For Tiffany, home is a place where many people know where to find her. She entertains and holds court from her favourite living room perch, and she offers her living room to many co-operative groups from which to plan events and happenings. Within her busy home, Tiffany has created places of quiet and reflection where she spends time painting, listening to her music, or contemplating the world.

We are still very much in the process of understanding and supporting people to define home. Two last images show how the people will tell us what we need to know if only we slow down and listen to what they are telling us.

Late at night when Brenda can't sleep, she gets dressed and sits down in the lobby. People often tell her Mom or a support person about this the next day. We were concerned about this until the stories grew a little bit. We realized that people would see Brenda on the in-house lobby cameras (broadcast onto their televisions), and invariably one, two or more people would come down and talk to her, sometimes invite her for tea, and most often walk her home and see her inside after awhile.

Matthew at two years old is a curious boy. One day when his mother is talking in the lobby, he jumps into an open elevator and the door closes. Donna calmly watches which floor it goes to and takes the next elevator up. Some neighbours are anxious and a bit critical about Donna's lack of fluster and concern. A few minutes later, she finds him on the fourth floor, knocking on his beloved neighbour, Tee's, door. She says to the flustered group in the lobby a few minutes later, "It's Rougemount. He just went to Theresa's door that he knows. What could happen to him here?"

These images belong in the later years and have helped us to understand the deep emotional level at which people have come to view their home as a safe and good place to live. What is a shock and needs a moment's adjustment within ourselves—this vulnerable person is out there and alone—has become second nature to Brenda and Donna. They feel the safety and the caring of the community that they are now a part. For us, at times, it can be an intellectual experience backed up with some good stories and experiences. For them, it is a lived experience.

If home is the first place and from it other good things can happen, then people are telling us that home is a very good place indeed. It sets the stakes high for the other parts of life: new relationships and a greater sense of community space and belonging.

Let me live
in a place of hope
where—
in the middle of imperfection—
potential runs deep
and possibility strong.

Let me grow
in a garden of wonder
where I am nourished
by hands of many colours
and guided by hands of many shapes.

Let me become
in a space of my own
where I can soar
protected by others
who hold me safe.

Let this be
that community of hope,
that abundant garden,
that space secure…

…and let me call it…home.

(Janet Klees, written for Rougemount's
tenth anniversary celebration)

Chapter 4
Tending to Relationship

In a world of technology, consumerism, and quick solutions, the families of Deohaeko are firm believers in the long, hard, uncertain work of embracing old fashioned, one-to-one relationships. People involved in personal, committed relationships stand by family members as human service systems rise and fall, elected bodies come and go, and typical human crises ebb and flow.

There was a powerful, tragic demonstration of this truth during the huge electrical black out which covered much of southern Ontario and northeastern United States in August of 2003. A young man had been disabled in a workplace accident two years prior and was living in a Toronto high rise apartment. He appeared to have all of current technology's bells and whistles to enable him to live a full life despite the loss of his legs and one arm, and the limitations imposed by his skin unable to regulate his temperature without air conditioning. His insurance program paid for the latest in physical technology—a completely adapted apartment, wheelchair, computers, and an adapted van. It also paid for advanced human service technology with assistants for personal support, home support and chauffeurs. His parents lived far away in northern Ontario, and he was a young man living the typical technology-assisted life others could only have dreamed about years ago.

However, when the lights went out, so did the young man's air conditioning and his lifeline to sustaining adequate body temperature. At the same time, all of the physical and human service technology failed him as well. Telephones did not work, elevators in his building did not function, automatic apartment doors could not function, emergency back ups failed, and assistants failed to arrive for work to support him. His parents tried frantically from hundreds of miles away but were unable to contact a single human soul to check on their son. And in the city of 3 million, with all of the technology in failure, there was not one real person who walked the seventeen flights of stairs to his apartment and battered down the door to save his life. No one within walking distance knew this young man well enough to think of lending a hand. The young man died that night for the lack of one human being person ready and able to put him first during that night of calamity.

For people connected with Deohaeko, when the lights went out, there were other people. At Rougemount, Don, a single, older man who is a cheerful neighbour of Donna and Matthew, was happy to find the only place in the neighbourhood with gas stoves to make him a Chinese take-out dinner. He was hungry, but saved over half of it and brought it over to Donna and Matthew to make sure they had some food for the night. He found them settled into the outside play area where most of the families with young children had gathered.

Brenda was with her neighbour, Hilda, when the lights went out. This reassured her that the problem was not hers alone. Her Supporter—a local woman who could walk the distance if necessary—made it in for the evening despite the uncertainty and then two neighbours checked in to make sure she was alright. Later, her mother arrived to stay the night and she felt safe and secure.

Family members, neighbours and Supporters arrived to check on Rob and Jon and John.

Outside of Rougemount, Caroline Ann was at the store when the blackout came, and she came home to family and friends who eventually gathered in the back yard to play cards and have a neighbourhood barbecue. Tiffany and her mom were met by her father and brought in from the airport after the last flight in from Halifax. Tiffany was invited to spend the next day at the home of a Supporter whose house was near the cooling breezes off the lake.

It was people who made each of these individuals feel safe and secure. Not only the people who personally rose to the occasion, but also the many, many people who called on available lines just to check for themselves that people were okay. It was also people in relationship with individuals who have a disability who made decisions and choices ten years ago when Rougemount was being built. Based on the value they placed on the presence of their sons and daughters in the life of the community, and therefore on all people, they ensured that Rougemount, in the event of power failure, would be a safe place. They planned for and installed generator power to light all the hallways and work the two elevators. This was not done by bureaucratic standards at the government level, or professional standards by architects or builders, but by people in relationship with vulnerable individuals.

And for the rest, it was personal relationships between individual people which made the difference during a hot summer blackout and continues to make a profound difference in the lives of people time and again.

So our faith is placed heavily upon relationship. Sure, the technology and the money for paid support form important parts of the whole picture for people with disabilities, but we have seen technology fail and we have seen human services fail. I think that the network of human relationships does not experience full system failure in the same way. While any given relationship might fail, the nature of complex relationships often means that they rarely fail all at the same time. When any of us allows and invites a full range of relationship into our lives, one or two 'light bulbs' may go out—a friend or family member may move away, die, or change, but there are others still there to move in and provide comfort and support. There seems to be an innate ability for many of these complex webs of relationship to repair themselves, to recognize gaps and weaknesses and invite others in to return to strength.

People who have a disability in our society are often seen as less than and different by most others in the society. They are stereotyped in negative ways that deny their unique gifts and devalue their presence in our midst. Shunned, rejected, and set aside (even with good intentions), people lead lives that run outside of the valued core of our society. Often they live separately (as in group homes), work separately (as in workshops) or not at all, and recreate separately (as in special and separate sports programs). As a group this makes them vulnerable to further poor treatment, further setting apart, and further situations that can put their very lives at risk. Most people in society do not come to know them as unique human beings who have a contribution to make to the greater community. Instead, people easily agree to substandard lives for those faceless people whom they do not know.

What can best protect the vulnerability of people at the edges of society is, ironically, the very thing from which they are separated—ordinary citizens. The vulnerability of people with a disability and their subsequent devaluation in our society can mean that the lifelong exercise of building, repairing and rebuilding a web of relationships in which we all learn to engage is denied to them. We need to figure out how to re-engage people in a difficult world. The words of Jean Vanier in *Becoming Human* give us a hopeful starting point:

Each person, big or small, has a role to play in the world. As we start to really get to know others, as we begin to listen to each other's stories, things begin to change. We no longer judge each other according to concepts of power and knowledge or according to group identity, but according to these personal, heart-to-heart encounters. We begin the movement from exclusion to inclusion, from fear to trust, from closedness to openness, from judgment and prejudice to forgiveness and understanding. It is a movement of the heart. We begin to see each other as brothers and sisters in humanity. We are no longer governed by fear, but by the heart. (p. 83)

The beginning of our hope stems from a deeper understanding that the building of relationship with vulnerable people is a gift for us all. We are not just doing it 'for' or 'to' someone else, we are doing it for ourselves.

And so, along with our ideas of making home and establishing valued presence in community, we also spend time and reflection on how to help individuals enter into this very human enterprise of building, experimenting with, repairing and rebuilding that safety web of relationships that will make life better for us all.

We have done so mainly, but not solely, by developing and sustaining circles of support with each vulnerable person. We find that having a circle is a simple way of holding one's faith and hope in the potential of relationship. It is a good idea to ask yourselves wherein you place your hope. Is it in a good human service, or in finding enough support dollars, or is it latching onto the right combination of drugs to alter behaviour? For us, the answer lies in people—people who will stand by and who will take action from a place of love and understanding over time. We have found that if our answer is, indeed, that we place our hope in people, then circles of support are one good way to hold people together. A circle can help people come together in a common understanding of the dreams, hopes, possible futures, current life, problems, fears, and what's been tried that surround one person and their family. Through the telling of old stories and working on new stories a common caring will develop. And through each meeting together, common experience can provide the people with strong bonds to move forward.

> To survive effectively in a fragmented society with little room for people with developmental disabilities, friends need to make a conscious choice to situate their friendship within a community of resistance.
>
> John O'Brien, Members of Each Other

It is with a bit of trepidation that I am including some of our stories and discoveries about circles at all in this book. Too often, good ideas or frameworks are latched onto as the definitive solution. Let me state from the start that *circles are not the answer.* They are not the answer to *any* question that you might ask. They are not the answer to how to find a good place to live for your son or daughter. They are not the answer to how to make sure that your family member is an active and welcome participant in her community. They are not the answer to making sure that your loved one is not isolated and lonely. They are not the answer to my fears of who will replace you when you are gone.

However, many people and organizations act as if circles are the answer to the woes that our often-uncaring society allows to be unanswered.

It has become very popular to hear people presenting and talking about circles at conferences. Many organizations are adopting policy statements that require that vulnerable people of all kinds have a circle. Funders' ears perk up when proposals include promises to build and sustain circles. In crisis, people are often asked, "yes, but did she have a circle?" Stories abound of circle successes, circle failures, and circle issues. Conferences are held about starting circles, recruiting for circles, barriers to circles and offer tips and solutions to common circle problems. Old organizations looking for new mandates and territory begin to offer services to help families develop circles. New organizations begin which promise to help families build circles to protect the future, or which promise to support your circle in the future when you are no longer there.

These are not necessarily bad things. People have indeed used the ideas of circles as a way of safeguarding individuals' lives, offering alternatives, fulfilling dreams, and moving on with ones' life. What becomes worrisome is when a person, an organization, a policy or a funder acts as if the circle, in and of itself, is a service or a technology or a tool which will automatically provide workable solutions to the individual and his or her situation. So when a person has lost a job, or wants a home, or feels lonely and isolated, they are given a circle. Or, rather are given a visit from a staff person who does not have the resources to find them a job, or a home, or a friend, but pledges to find family members and volunteers and other staff who will form a circle and meet every month with that individual. After many months, the person may not yet have the job, the home, or the friends, and may not even have a circle with any genuine relationships. The real needs of the individual are held at bay. This is a circle used as a tool, a technology, the latest 'fix' which promises to, but will not, make sure that the individual lives a good life. The difference between this kind of circle and the old provincially mandated Individual Program Planning since the 1980s is negligible.

Such examples are doomed to failure. Circles cannot and will not take the place of members of society who work hard to listen, understand and come to personally care about a person and their circumstances.

A circle is simply one kind of way of holding and shaping the work, the thought, the caring, and the people that are the only ingredients that matter in whatever set of 'solutions' are decided upon. In such a circle, when a person loses their job, they are likely to call a friend, who is a part of the circle of important relationships that keep the person well, and meet them for lunch and work out a way to apply for another job, rather than to wait for or call a circle meeting and figure it out with the whole group. It's not the circle who answers the phone or suggests lunch. It's not the circle who hears about another opportunity and figures it out with the person. It is another person—a person who has come to know and listen to the one who has lost a job. The circle is the place that these two people are linked with a number of like-minded others to move in a common direction. The circle is one way to hold and invite relationship.

What Others Say

A great blessing for the families of Deohaeko is to be in an area of the world where many people are actively exploring and experimenting with various ideas about circles—their strengths, their boundaries and limitations, and their varying arrangements. We have learned from many other families in Durham region who use circles to bring relationship more securely into their own and their family member's lives. Some families do so on their own, some are linked with other families in small groups somewhat similar to ours, and some are loosely linked to encouraging agencies, or a newly-forming provincial body, *Lifetime Circles*. Learning events and time spent with Peter Dill, John O'Brien, Darcy Elks and others have strengthened our thinking and our experiences.

We have been strongly affected by the powerful potential of an effective circle. We have come to understand that the best circles have something to do with listening well and with heart, something to do with personal commitment, something to do with inviting and welcoming as old-fashioned community virtues, something to do with taking thoughtful action, something to do with mutuality, and a lot to do with determination and perseverance in the face of adversity.

John O'Brien has been helpful in assisting us not to make our circles too rigid. He says that:

> *Families need containers for their dreams. What is useful about a container is its emptiness, its openness to be filled with what a family really wants. This useful emptiness can be made through the experience of belonging to a web of personal support especially when that broad web of relationships becomes deep and dense as people gather to listen, to share, to shape a powerful way of understanding and to act on their world. (pp. 22-23 in Tell Me a Story of Deep Delight)*

John further illustrates his ideas with three stanzas from the *Tao Te Ching*:

> *We join spokes together in a wheel,*
> *But it is the centre hole*
> *That makes the wagon move.*
> *We shape clay into a pot,*
> *But it is the emptiness inside*
> *That holds whatever we want.*
> *We hammer wood for a house,*
> *But it is the inner space*
> *That makes it liveable.*
>
> Tao Te Ching in John O'Brien's
> *Tell Me a Story of Deep Delight)*

Peter Dill says that a circle is a journey and the invitation to a journey. It is a place for people to tell their stories and a place for people to dream. This is important in a world where the impact of systems is the loss of dreams and of dreaming. Circles live on the edge of systems. They must do so because listening to the hearts of people must be ever flexible. (*Friends for Life, 2002, p. 3*)

Bruce Uditsky underlines our thinking about not turning making friends into a technology. He has written powerfully on *Natural Pathways to Friendship* where he states that it is important to stay with natural ways of entering into friendship in these times of professionalism and technology aimed at things that are human. There are no simple solutions to complex human problems. There is, however, the option to look at the ways in which people have naturally always entered into friendship. When we do this we recognize great potential for following the same kinds of pathways together with a person with a disability. Such natural pathways may include meeting through mutual friends, sharing a common experience, seeking out familiar places, being of similar age, culture or neighbourhood, sharing common interests sharing common struggles, and being together out of necessity.

This kind of thinking underscores our initial impulse not to use circles as a uniform way to "help people get friends and relationships in their lives". We try to think about helping individuals to meet people and enter into relationships as key, and as circles (in the ways Peter Dill and John O'Brien talk about them) as one helpful way to bring together some of the people and the thinking that might help us get there.

What We've Learned Through and With Circles

Early on in Deohaeko history, we decided that we needed to find out how to help make home with people who had never done so and who were generally not expected to do so in any real or significant way during their lifetime. In much the same way, we came to understand and take on the task of building strong, flexible and personal relationship networks with people who had lost many of the formative years and typical experiences upon which most of us begin building our relationships. Circles have been a good way for the families and friends of Deohaeko to learn good lessons about building relationship.

Circles, when they work fairly well, are the place in which people can begin to experience the belonging, the mutuality and the magic of relationship first hand. People can learn some valuable lessons about relationship with their circle, and about faith and trust and dreaming. In a world where relationship is the number one safeguard, circles may offer a beginning place for relationship to take place.

As I write I worry that many readers will skim through the introductory paragraphs, and settle on the experiences of our group. These items will then be added to their list of ingredients for their own "recipe for circle development". The recipe will not work. It will lead to people no longer seeing the possibility of circles, to funders not funding work related to circles, and eventually to individuals being hurt and deceived in the name of circles.

Circles will not guarantee results—relationship or otherwise. However, with thought and care, a circle may be an opportunity for people to come together and explore and rediscover some of the gifts of relationship. A circle is just one way to do so, but in this world of technology, the ways of the past are fast disappearing and maybe a few circles will help a wider range of ordinary citizen recapture the meaning and heart of one-to-one relationship.

Over the past eight years, we have worked hard at thinking about circles in many different ways. Today we know much more about the possibility of circles, their potential and also their limitations.

Eight years ago, we were at a time when all individuals were involved in a circle of some kind. These circles seemed to work well enough for some of the things we were working on at the time—helping people to establish home, finding jobs and work, maintaining a presence in the community. Since then, as we have turned to a focus on meaningful community connections and developing deep relationship we have had to look at our circles in new ways.

Our Circles are Not Perfect

All of our circles are imperfect and need constant energy and attention. Our work and attention to building, maintaining and re-working our circles has led us to some wonderful places. At the same time, we struggle greatly with our day-to-day challenges. Some of these challenges include the following.

Donna's circle has been especially wonderful at times that have called for intensity and commitment, like during her pregnancy, her baby's first few months, and the death of her mother. But we worry that the circle consists of several Deohaeko members at the very core, and very busy others just beyond that. It will need to share the accountability across newer members if it is to move well into the future.

Brenda stopped having regular circle times because they felt too Supporter-driven. Some of the new formats have been very hopeful, but we have not re-gained the momentum of regular meeting times. Jon's full circle rarely meets because it is so hard to find common meeting times. Large annual gatherings help somewhat, but a dedicated core needs to get together more often. A meeting of Supporters happens more regularly, but we know this is not a circle. It has become clear to us that John does not like the group meeting and talking aspect of most circle times. These have been phased out in exchanged for very casual living room conversations, but we feel that important people are being left out. Tiffany's circle meets regularly but we struggle to have the same friends and neighbours come out each time. The continuity is hard to maintain. At the same time, Tiffany holds wonderful annual events such as a summer barbecue and a Christmas Tree Trimming Tea that remind everyone how good it is to be together. Rob's circle gatherings are very regular and good information and planning happens. However, despite many attempts to increase circle membership the group remains very small.

Some newer events lead us to hope once again that this may change. Caroline Ann's circle has had some great ebb and flow. At times, Caroline Ann's circle has been large, lively and creative, effectively working together in many ways. It has also struggled with people losing commitment or being led away by the rest of their lives. Recouping has been a struggle.

This list is not meant to discourage families from beginning a circle, but as a way to say that even with the struggles such as those outlined above, we have achieved some of the wonderful things described below. Struggle is just a part of life.

Not Everything Happens Within the Circle

Life is busy and it is complex. It would be contrived and constraining to require that all decisions made and new directions enacted through the circle. Circles tend to meet on a fairly regular basis, but never often enough to meet the spontaneity and speed with which we need to make decisions about our lives. So, outside of our circle gatherings, for each person, much of life happens. When a person takes on a new work or volunteer role in the community, they begin to meet and develop new relationships with others. It is usually not the right moment to begin to invite such new people to circle gatherings. Interactions with neighbours might be positive and genuine, but this may not be the person to be invited to circle gatherings, either.

Circle members collectively hold the picture of the person's life in their hands, hearts and minds. However the circle gathering can only deal with one piece of it at a time. Sometimes the circle instigates. Sometimes, it broadens and deepens the issues at hand. Sometimes it trouble shoots and problem solves. Sometimes it reacts and judges events and roles in play.

Essentially, circle times might capture a moment in time of a person's life and members are able to react to, plan and think ahead from that moment (based on previous history and experience, of course). This is the time to reflect, enjoy past and current successes, deepen our understanding, make plans for some of the time ahead, ensure that the individual continues to have a voice about her life, and enjoy the relationships among circle members present. We have little time for such oases of reflection, renewal and true community in our busy lives. There is great value in these gatherings for these reasons. In between circle times, the rest of life happens in its haphazard, rushed and ever-changing form.

Learning to Listen

Caroline Ann began to tell us in many ways that she was not fully happy in her Rougemount home about two years before her true dreams of home were realized. At first, friends and family both outside of and within her circle, thought she was requesting small changes be made to deepen her sense of home. We diligently made plans to involve Caroline Ann in some additional roles in the co-operative office to increase her sense of belonging and purpose. We helped her move from the front of the building to a quieter apartment facing the back in order to meet her concerns for fire truck sirens that would pass her windows. We worked hard at a relationship within the building that would occasionally give her great stress. We tried to maximize visits with her sister Barbara and new nephew Terry. We talked about Caroline Ann moving to the first floor in order to have immediate access to the outside gardens. At some point, however, a courageous and sensitive circle member being consulted about priorities for circle discussion said, "what Caroline Ann really wants to talk about is actually moving out of Rougemount and into another place to call home."

At that moment, I learned that strong, vibrant circles help people enter into relationship with others, and when effective, they listen in order to bring about the changes that are yearned. This is not as easy as it sounds. John O'Brien talks about "listening with an open heart" but we are quick to judge and offer what we think is right or good.

We, in Caroline's circle, came to learn to listen to the yearnings of her heart. We listened and tried to put aside our mixed emotions—sadness that Rougemount was not able to be home for her, excitement that we were on a new and uncharted path together, fear that we would fail her in this bid altogether, worry that there would be so many new questions ahead.

Caroline's mother, Helen, talks about that time in a different way. "I think that I knew ahead of others that Caroline Ann would need to move, and slowly it came to me that a move back to our family home, in her own separate apartment would be a good move. I had some concerns about voicing this option because it might be seen by others as a step back. At the same time I felt the exhilaration of doing the right thing for the whole family— Caroline Ann would be newly returned to the very midst of our family—always for those spontaneous moments. That felt right."

Learning to Walk With Donna

The story of Donna's circle which she has drawn around herself and little Matthew is one to be told. It is so rich with the various perspectives and the joys and difficulties all at the same time. At the same time, it is a story of learning to walk with a woman whose life is her very own.

Donna was just turning 30, when she told us she was having a baby. In retrospect, this should not have been a surprise, but it was because most of Donna's circle members thought that we had a pretty good handle on the events and priorities in her life. Indeed we did—sort of. We were, in fact, all very clear that Donna dearly wanted to be married and have a family of her own. To that end, we were all frustrated by our lack of success in introducing her to the sort of men who might help make this dream become a reality. However, we did not count on Donna making the sort of conclusions that many women seem to make these days and decide that if she were to wait for the right guy to come along, she might have to give up the dream of having a baby altogether. Furthermore, no one counted on Donna deciding on involving no one but herself in this important, life-defining decision. Her way was clear, and she could imagine what range of conditions might be put in her way if this came to be a group decision.

All of our personal values, beliefs and ideas were put to the test. Could we help Donna walk the path she had so clearly chosen? It took discussion, prayer and a wise and welcoming grandmother to help us focus on the wonder of the events: a child would be born. And we would all hold him in the embrace of our love and caring for Donna and Marje to make sure that his life was as right and good as Donna's. It was a challenge and a test.

Eight women stood up to the test—a combination of other Deohaeko parents, friends, and Supporters. Together, we figured out the medical issues, the baby supplies, and social assistance implications. We figured out how to provide the one-to-one learning that would help Donna best to learn the many things that lay ahead. We used ourselves, friends, and family. In the end, we even helped Donna to hire a doula, (a woman specifically trained to provide care for new moms and babies after birth). The doula, too, became part of our group and has stayed on for the three years since!

Suddenly, 'walking with' Donna had less to do with circle discussions, planning, implementing solid plans and evaluating the aftermath. Walking with had to do with a baby arriving in 4 months and what to do about medical check ups, her congenital heart condition, the size of her apartment, and finding all the right baby stuff! 'Walking with' had to include listening carefully and hearing the joy and excitement in Donna and helping organize an impromptu 'Celebration of Life' party within the co-operative. Walking with Donna was a matter of thinking through Children's Aid Society concerns and the baby's best interests, and coming to firmly believe that Donna could be a good mother with guidance and support. We worked through a complex after-birth support plan. Donna was, of course, front and centre of every decision and every plan that we built. Then, we met with the CAS so effectively that the record shows that "There is no role for CAS in this situation".

Donna entered a downtown city hospital at the highest possible level 'high risk pregnancy' care program available, and was immediately labelled 'mentally handicapped'. She nonetheless forced an unsuspecting team of doctors and nurses to radically change their perceptions of what this label might mean. She and three circle members (including proud Grandma, of course) worked through a planned induction where Donna was later described by hospital staff as "grace under fire", and managed a completely natural delivery of a fine 7 pound 12 ounce baby boy. Donna then went on to stay for a full six days on the ward, fully supported by family and circle members at all times, to work hard at establishing breast feeding with constant assistance from an admiring staff ("If only all of the Moms here would work this hard at getting it started!").

We also learned to deal with the unexpected. To Donna's delight, her sister-in-law who lives out of town, came to stay with Donna for the first week home. While this was mostly very positive for Donna and Matthew, it came with some unexpected curves for Donna and her circle. It became clear, that due to distance, time and perspective, our way of organizing and supporting was not familiar to this family member. It took some time for the sister-in-law to trust the complex arrangement of supports that the circle had arranged for Donna, and some time for the circle to move back from these plans during her visit. It took a fair bit of time after that visit, for the circle to fully re-instate their original plans and for Donna to feel comfortable with those plans again. We all learned that family is important. Circle members are important. When time, distance and circumstance do not bring these two together we need to create bridges and ways for people to trust each other to work effectively together in times of need (usually the only times when they might come together). Walking with Donna opened us to honouring chosen family that we had not yet come to know.

Today, Matthew is an active, engaging, loving little boy. Donna works hard at keeping up with all of his new skills and demands, as all parents do. At this time, Erin, her doula, spends about three visits every week with Donna, one of those is attending the local YMCA Child Drop In program. Often, Erin manages to bring her own three-year old son along. She also helps Donna with planning and learning to prepare healthy meals and snacks, with planning her time and her money, and with coping through Matthew's childhood illnesses.

Other circle members have taken on other roles. One member offers rides and company when Donna wants to take Matthew to the doctor unexpectedly (she goes a bit more often than many because she does not want to make a mistake around his health). Another member drops by regularly to help out with whatever is going on—a bath for Matthew, watching Matthew so Donna can throw some laundry in, figuring out a healthy snack, or getting Matthew outside to play.

After a period of focused searching, we also managed to introduce Donna and a young mother who lives about 20 minutes away and who now spends some spontaneous, fun 'mom' time with Donna and Matthew. This new friendship provides Donna with a new outlook on family, raising children, and being a home-based Mom.

At the co-operative, Matthew knows many people well, and happily spends time with one neighbour or another when Donna needs to attend a co-operative meeting. He loves to play with the other kids in the hallways. He adores his Uncle Bob, who gives him treats and returns his affection quietly.

Matthew is a bright and happy three-year old who is truly a child of the Rougemount community. Donna is his proud, ever-learning, competent mother but in the way of her true nature she shares him unstintingly with all members who reach out to him. We have learned a lot in three years. Our expectations of Donna have been stretched time and time again. We have had to all stretch ourselves in building good life situations for both mother and child, but we have done it well and all feel a sense of accomplishment in this achievement. By walking with Donna and not telling her what to do, we have re-discovered how a community might work together to raise a child.

A Circle is Not a Focus Meeting

For Tiffany, when some members come together every six weeks or so, it is called a focus meeting. So for Tiffany and her family, the circle is not an event, but rather a description of the web of relationships in Tiffany's life. Some of the people who make up that circle may be invited to a focus meeting but many others would be unable to come. The members who come for the focus meeting are used to help the day's discussion evolve, to raise relevant issues, to brainstorm ideas. These members, who may substantially but not completely change from meeting to meeting, help to hold the vision of Tiffany's life but they are not alone. Typically, the people who seem to make it to the focus meeting are people who live in the co-operative, close family members (mother, father), Deohaeko members, one or two current Supporters, and friends of long-standing who live near by. Other people are considered important people in Tiffany's life, but cannot make it to focus meetings most of the time. These people are still a part of her web of support. They include her two aunts and uncle in Nova Scotia, her father's family in Belleville, a most recent roommate of five years, the rest of the Deohaeko Support Network, at least ten or more Rougemount neighbours who know Tiffany well, one or two neighbours from her old neighbourhood, a couple of previous Supporters.

Tiffany's Circle: *the people to hold the vision of a life that Tiffany wishes to have...*

...to listen with heart
...to deepen the dreams with understanding
...to brainstorm the details with joy
...to evaluate and re-work the outcomes with love

Learning to See the Circle

Being part of the experience of Tiffany's circle, we learned to see the web of relationships rather than just a meeting. This was valuable to us as we became very involved with learning how to truly see Donna's evolving circle.

In the winter of 2002-2003, Donna's mother, Marje discovered that she had bone and lung cancer and she probably had three months to live. She was visiting her older son in Ingersoll at the time and it was subsequently decided not to move her back to Pickering. This was a difficult decision for Donna and her brother Bob, also of

Rougemount, to live with and manage. Donna's recognized circle at the time essentially included now eleven women who had supported her through the birth of Matthew and their first two years together. The task ahead of us was demanding. We need to figure out meaningful ways for Donna and Matthew to spend quality time with Marje in a hospital setting in an unfamiliar town, more than two hours away.

Tiffany's experience allowed me to sit down and really contemplate the next evolution of Donna's circle. Slowly, it became clear to me that it was not I, or even the current circle who was re-inventing this web of relationships. It was clearly a process in which Donna was the dynamic centre. I only had to recognize it. I asked myself: who are the people to whom Donna is reaching out in her grief and distress and from whom she is able to derive some comfort.

To varying degrees all of the Deohaeko families were on this list, as were her two support persons. Important others who came forward included Gaytri, a co-operative member with two young sons who provided many cups of tea, a listening ear, and a solid co-operative presence. Arlene, a previous co-operative member and neighbour to Donna and Marje, came forward to look after Matthew, call and talk with Donna, reminisce about Marje. Bob, her brother, was there in new and very supportive ways for Donna and Matthew and began to be very much involved in day-to-day ways. Cathy, Donna's fairly new friend who was also a young mother provided lots of listening time, some get away with the kids time, and some babysitting while Donna was in Ingersoll. Theresa, who lives in the building and is a long-time friend, was there at all times. Pat was always there to answer questions. Kathy, a friend from school days began to visit more regularly and sometimes stayed over during a long night. Many other co-operative members were clearly there for Donna at all times. Donna held a candle light vigil when her Mom was in the hospital. She held a luncheon together with the families of Deohaeko after the funeral. She recently held a small tea in memory of her mother's birthday. To each of these events came a solid, dedicated number of neighbours and friends (from 10 to over 60 people per event) who stood by to pray, add memories, provide affirmation, and offer support. This is a brief outline of Donna's web of support. I am only grateful that I learned to see it.

On a smaller scale, we have learned to look for and see the circles of support that reach out to people on a daily basis. I am reminded of a Wednesday afternoon a few years ago, when Brenda had been having a rough week—dental surgery, discomfort from eating too many bananas another day, and an upset with a Supporter which could not be well resolved in her mind because the Supporter was sick the next day. By Wednesday, Brenda was disgruntled and pacing out on her first floor patio, unhappy with her world. Across the parking lot a few neighbours sat at the picnic table under the maple tree, and noticed her. "Come and join us," encouraged Ann, Jean, Bob and Barb. Brenda didn't reply but someone saw a small smile while she hesitated in her pacing. Barb suddenly asked Brenda if she could come in and use her washroom. Brenda agreed, and when Barb returned, Brenda followed her outside. That was at 1:30 in the afternoon. She was still there talking and laughing under the trees an hour and a half later. At 4:00, she walked inside with the last neighbour remaining.

What is important to understand that when Brenda was low and upset, she ended up spending an afternoon with friends and left feeling better. Neighbours noticed her distress and responded to her natural and caring ways. No one thought to call 'staff' or family to solve a problem that was not theirs. They simply saw a neighbour feeling low and believed that their invitation to join them would be a comfort. They even persisted in finding a creative way (asking to use her washroom) for Brenda to join them when a simple invitation did not work. This does not make them the close, intimate circle members who help Brenda with the large decisions in her life, but it does mean that there are supportive people around her who take part in helping her live well and feel safe and included.

This aspect of community life was captured in one of the early Rougemount Friday news sheets in a small musing written by Linda Dawe.

> Communities are Circles of People. Sometimes these circles overlap. When people are gathered around a common purpose you see the meaning of life: people talking to one another, joking as they get tired, helping each other, caring for one another. What is most valuable about this is that it creates community where it doesn't matter at all what you earn, how you dress, what your politics are, you just work and laugh together anyhow.

We believed that this could happen and that it would happen. What was new was learning to *see* it happen in very ordinary ways.

Trying Out Ways to Include Sisters and Brothers

Rob has two brothers and a sister. The other three are married and have young, busy children and full work lives. They live some distance from Rob's home. Rob's formal circle, which meets regularly is small and at times, seems somewhat resistant to efforts to grow. Harriet and Orest have spent some time thinking about this, and have tried some interesting variations to include Rob's busy brothers, sister, nieces and nephews in his life. They felt that Rob was busy and contributing in his own meaningful ways, and that the typical family gatherings were inadequate for anyone to truly understand Rob and his current life. One attempt to change this is referred to by Orest as the "mobile circle". Since these young families' lives were filled with activities, schedules and responsibilities that did not allow for a regular participation in the formal circle, Rob would come to them.

So, on Saturdays for a few months, Rob began to make the tour of his brothers and sister's homes. He brought photo albums and information outlining what his week and time looked like. A Supporter who knew him well and could assist in talking about Rob and his life accompanied him. He was also to spend some time on his own with his brothers and sister and their spouses and children so they could know him more personally than at family gatherings.

This mobile circle was a short-term effort that spanned several months. It has helped us to identify the problems that distance, young family life, and full time jobs can have on developing typical relationships among sisters and brothers. It has helped to see that Rob's inclusion in family gatherings only develops a certain level of intimacy and relationship and that a different approach is needed for a different level of relationship. Finally, it has caused us to recognize the vital role that a Supporter might play in these visits and in developing these relationships. The Supporter must be friendly and outgoing without taking over. He must be a model of respectful support (words, manner, topics of conversation) for the sister or brother. He is teaching by his very presence and attitude. He must be able to convey information but do so in such a way that the sister or brother do not worry that their own support will not be specialized enough. This work requires a very sensitive Supporter and much pre-planning.

Another recent attempt at including sisters and brothers and their families was the planning of a Sunday afternoon tea and open house in the beautiful Big Room at Rougemount overlooking a part of the Rouge Valley. Harriet and Orest, together with Supporters, put together large, themed photographic displays outlining Rob's interests, roles, and current involvements, including the friends, neighbours and acquaintances that he encountered during his week. Family, friends, neighbours and acquaintances were all invited. Although the turnout of newer acquaintances from the community was lower than

Harriet and Orest had hoped, Rob's sister, brothers, nieces, nephews and cousins came out in full force. Their interest, surprise and admiration for Rob's achievements were plain to see. They learned a lot about him that day. They learned from the themed posters which depicted him so actively involved in valued ways in the whole community. They learned from the other 30 or so neighbours and friends who came by and obviously knew some aspect or other of Rob so marvellously well. And they learned from Rob himself, in his obvious delight of being in the midst of so many familiar faces.

Learning to Harness the Energy and Potential of the Larger Circle

Jon and his family also found it difficult to bring the many people who know and care about Jon into his circle on a regular basis. As an alternate approach, we decided to invite a wide range of people who know Jon in some capacity to join us for an evening gathering in order for Jon's parents to talk about his life and to help others begin to think about the bigger issues in Jon's life. We have since gathered such a group together three times for Jon. The first time was around his 21st birthday and was an invitation to help figure out work options in these transition years. The other times were more to remind participants of the importance of relationship to Jon, to give them some details about parts of his life with which they were not familiar, and to think of deepening some of his roles.

The people to respond to these invitations have included: Jon's sister and two aunts, Jon's grandmother (and grandfather to one event before he passed away), neighbours from his old neighbourhood, friends of his sister, co-operative neighbours, his small business customers, family members of a farm he stays at from time to time, family members of supporters, past teachers, past Supporters, and Rougemount neighbours.

These gatherings have been helpful and practical in several ways. The quality of the ideas and brainstorming, with resulting contacts and connections has been wonderful. Due to the wide range of people who—typically 20-25 people attend—the discussions about typical expectations and dreams for young men in Durham Region have been full and genuine.

The gatherings have increased the information that people have about Jon. Although the information is not very detailed and is not first hand, it at least allows people to imagine what Jon's life currently looks like. It motivates a few people to ask more questions and get to know him a little bit better.

Perhaps most importantly, this format allows us to bring up the larger context of Jon's life. We have been able to talk about planning work options with Jon, by looking to what other young men are doing in the area. This helps to ensure that this is the measure by which we gauge success in his life—not by looking at what other disabled young men might be doing, which is a different comparison altogether. We have been able to stress the importance of relationship in Jon's life. We have been able to hold up a standard of the kind of home life, choices, control, work and recreation that Jon now enjoys. While there are still many areas to fill in better ways, this large group of people, all in all, have a very positive view of what Jon's life is like. We can only hope this is a standard that they will strive to maintain over time.

The other benefit of this form of gathering is that it is a community kind of event. People like to come. Their ideas are welcomed and they feel good about contributing to make a difference. They are enriched by the experienced, I believe. That is one of the reasons that they returned to each of the three gatherings.

Learning to Take Support Issues Away from Circle Times

Brenda is a woman who makes her demands for a good life filled with genuine people clear in direct ways. Figuring out good support takes much time, energy, observation and guidance. Large challenges arise regularly and require discussion and common problem-solving. Brenda taught us that while such concerns are valid, and at times even vital, they do not belong in her circle.

We noticed that Brenda was becoming less involved in circle discussion, and in fact, would roam around her home for quite awhile before settling in to become part of the circle gathering. After some discussion, her mother Elizabeth and I thought a few things were going on. First of all, Brenda has a lot of support people in her life. They are all free to come to the circle, and even if half of them attend, they may constitute half of the group. Secondly, in their attempt to take part in the discussion, they often misunderstood the goal of the circle and raised their own issues for brainstorming or problem solving.

We are admittedly slow in our attempts to broaden the circle and outnumber the Supporters who attend. However, we felt that we could immediately address the second issue. We began to institute monthly Supporter meetings away from Brenda's apartment, and have the circles on the alternate month. At the same time, we started to let supporters know that when we meet for the circle, this is Brenda's time and as much as possible, she would decide what to talk about. This has led to much greater participation from Brenda. We have learned to be comfortable with lots of small talk, tea and waiting while Brenda figures out what kinds of things she would like to talk about that day. We have found she really wants to tell us about improvements that need to be made to her home, night disturbances that bother her sleep, and the kinds of things she has been doing with her time. She likes to talk about and remind us of her favourite people in the co-operative. She likes us to use the time to remind people that her journal (for communication) should read like a story of her week that she shares with her mother on the weekend. She likes to know that something good is going to happen for her at the end of the gathering time, so there is not a mass exodus and she is left on her own. These agenda are very different from the ones that we used to have. They are Brenda's and tell us a lot about what is important in her life.

No Cookie Cutter Circles

It doesn't have to look like a circle (whatever that is) to be a circle. Caroline Ann had several circle times in the cozy Member's Room in the co-operative before she moved, where her sister brought her beloved nephew, Terry, along and a friend, Sharon brought along her young son, William. Suddenly half of the circle was on the floor playing with babies, snacking and feeling very relaxed. The tone was very relaxed and Caroline Ann talked about many things quite easily when the main focus was no longer on her.

In an effort to include a few different people, we organized a tea at Brenda's park site in the late Fall. The Watershed Rehabilitation Project coordinator, Angie, came to join us as we sat on folding chairs, sipped tea and admired the view over the bay. To Brenda's delight we talked about nature and birds and things she knows about much more than we do within the confines of her apartment. A few months later, a slightly different group, including several neighbours and a couple of their children, gathered in Brenda's apartment to make Christmas decorations, eat goodies and chat.

These are not the typical ways that we think about circles, but the outcomes are solid enough for us to realize that we should not put circle formats into a box and expect wonderful things to happen. Although Brenda's gatherings do not yet constitute a conscious circle, they are an important beginning to having some new people in

Brenda's life see her in relaxed and positive ways, in a context in which she shines. These events remind us to find ways to allow the person to define the circle and not vice versa.

Not Letting Circles Get in the Way of Relationship

Caroline's circle has been meeting a lot less often lately. Typically, Caroline Ann calls to her a wonderfully diverse group of family, friends and neighbours. Focus meetings, as she calls them, are not always her favourite times, but people have worked on making them work for her. She is never put on the spot. We often meet at restaurants and make it a social occasion. The agenda flow from Caroline's life. For example, it was the members of her wide circle who managed to pull off a fantastic 40th birthday celebration one year. Another time a few members of the circles met in order to help out with a Supporter interview.

In speaking with Helen, Caroline's mother, about this latest development, she said to me that many of the most important people in Caroline's circle lead very busy lives and had limited time to devote to Caroline Ann on a regular basis. They were keen and they care greatly for Caroline, but in the stress of their daily lives they felt like they would rather spend some time alone doing something together with Caroline Ann than attending a focus meeting. Put that way, it seemed important not to let circles get in the way of relationships happening. Caroline's time is currently better occupied by having a number of dates with circle members, than it would be with one focus meeting attended by many members..

The circle still needs to meet. There are still important parts of joint discussion that need to get done. But this is the wise, temporary action of a mother who is sensitive to the priority of rhythms of relationship over formal circles.

Every Circle is a Learning and Teaching Moment

I have learned that there is no such thing as a circle gathering for which you do not prepare because it is easygoing or unimportant. You must always be prepared to address values and principles issues as they come up. During most circles there is little spontaneous time to address values issues as they come up. We often choose to talk about one chunk at a time, and in very practical ways. The concept of devaluation, which is very important to our understanding of why things are so and what we must do about it, can be initially dealt with in a few statements: *"As we know, society does not value or treat all of its members equally. Society tends to value speed, productivity, richness, beauty, newness. People who are not perceived to hold these qualities, or indeed are perceived to hold the opposite, are not valued. At a glance, this person is not seen by most of society as holding these qualities. We need to do something about this."* If such statements bring about discussion and debate, or arise a few times, we might plan to take a larger chunk of time in the future to have a fuller discussion.

In almost all circle gatherings, we find the occasion and take the opportunity to remind people to focus on two things—achieving the vision (working on positive roles and initiatives based on dreams and personal goals) and protecting vulnerabilities (decreasing negative roles and image issues). This is a chunk that can often be easily held by a group.

Occasionally, I will work with family members to provide a time during a circle meeting for a larger chunk of learning to happen. We might look at the life experiences of the person and the impact of those experiences on their current life, hopes and dreams. It might be focused on how to keep relationships front and centre of our thinking and our work (may be based on information in Chapter 7). It might be drawing out a visual diagram of current positive and negative roles that the person holds for a discussion of what to minimize, what to accentuate, and where to go next.

There are many opportunities within circle times to seize upon ideas that will help to focus all members on the various issues that support or suppress the building of relationships. Each five-minute discussion is an investment in our vision. These are some of the entry points that we have discovered:

- Supporters need to focus on their role—they are not the friend; they are the bridge to friendship with others.
- We cannot create friends, but we can build good opportunities in which friendships may flourish—we call this designing a context for relationship.
- Committed relationships will keep people safer than rules, laws, or policy.
- A chance to reflect on what all circle members gain from the person with a disability, followed by a talk on the mutuality of relationships.
- Where and how people typically find their friends. Make comparisons and design similar conditions for this person. Circle members who didn't think they have anything to offer begin to understand their role.
- How other circle members have helped this person to engage with others, encouraged friendships, etc.

Everything Matters Within a Circle Time

Everything counts. Everything tells a story to the participants. How you, the main family member, and others respond at every step of the way changes the course of action. We have found that serving a cup of tea and allowing time for chat and catching up is a good use of time at the beginning of most meetings. It sets the tone that the circle is about relationships more than it is about meetings.

We think about using time well in other ways, too. Take the time to tell stories. Tell old and well-loved tales to newcomers to the circle. Tell new stories with a bit of history to relate old and new achievements and events. This solidifies the roots of why we are looking for this kind of job, this kind of role, or this new hobby. Use the time to look at the person's week as a whole and teach how to evaluate it. Use the group to brainstorm all kinds of ideas. Brainstorm all the roles that typical 30-year old men hold in your region. Brainstorm all of the activities and relationships associated with being a gardener. Use the time to ask for all kinds of things that may be easy for circle members to provide: who can send her an e-mail once a month? Who can pop in while I am in Halifax next week? Who knows of anyone who might provide support on Monday nights to go to the gym? What can we do to celebrate her birthday next month?

The Circle Agenda Should Fit the Person and the Situation

When *The Tiffany Touch*, Tiffany's baking business, was in high gear the details of the business were not dealt with at focus meetings. The circle was informed about the general profile of the business, and certainly any new achievements. However, for effective decision-making we struck a four-person advisory group. This group was small enough to convene as needed and act quickly. In many respects this group acted to give direction to Tiffany's Supporter. Among other things the group was able to meet with a bank manager to understand more about business planning, to find an affordable, commercial-type kitchen, and to approve an intense pre-Christmas sale. It was also able to make the difficult decision to slow down the level of the business in light of poor profit prognosis (together with less time to fully involve Tiffany in enough aspects of the business).

This short-term advisory group was, in effect, a sub-circle for Tiffany's business. It was the right place for deeper discussion about decisions and direction. The creation of this group allowed the focus meetings to deal with the things that the people gathered could comment on or contribute to.

In a similar way, there are times in people's lives where important aspects must be dealt with but it is not comfortable or appropriate to do so within the whole circle. This happens when there are serious medical issues that may affect the parent, or when the parent is struggling with other serious issues in their lives. People who are especially close to the parent may meet in a much smaller grouping to try and figure out the implications for the son or daughter, personal support for the parent, and a myriad of other details.

Sometimes, the whole circle is too cumbersome or too complex to get together for all the decisions that need to be made. This past year with Donna's circle has shown us this. Donna needs someone to talk through many important decisions. When Marje was still alive, she took on the role of assisting with this daily decision-making. Now that the circle has come to fill her role, we have come to understand that it is impossible for us to meet as a group whenever decisions need to be made. Instead Donna figured out a way of talking to one of an inner core of five people who know the overall balance of her life well enough to help Donna make the decision. Circle times are then a time to update each other on news, to review bigger decisions, strengthen the ones that work, and troubleshoot the ones that don't.

The Circle Can Lead the Way in a Community That is Uncertain

When Donna let people know that she was having a baby, the reaction of the community was uncertain and mixed. Some people immediately started counselling her on abortion or adoption. Some people were worried about how her mother might view this event. Some people were happy that Donna was clearly so pleased to be having a child. Once Donna's circle gathered and talked with her about her plans and hopes and dreams, we really felt that she had a good chance to fulfil her dreams of motherhood. We also understood that the co-operative community seemed uncertain about how to respond to Donna. We decided to have a party for Donna and invite people to come and have a 'celebration of new life'. It turned out to be a wonderful way for neighbours and friends to come together and pledge their support for Donna and her baby. We found that once we had set the tone, most people responded to Donna with joy and good wishes. We also found the evening provided some neighbours a way to express their worries and concerns, which in turn provided us with ways to help them see that we did not ignore these practical issues, but had a plan in place for most of them. During that celebration, several people turned their concerns into a concrete offer of help. This also set the groundwork for concerns that arose over the following three years. People came to understand that there was a whole group of people looking out for this young family. Even today they bring concerns forward when they are still small enough to be easily addressed. They have become partners in keeping this family well.

Late in Donna's pregnancy, she received a call from the local Children's Aid Society, asking that she come down to their offices so they could assess her situation. Circle members quickly turned the invitation around so that a worker came and met Donna in her own apartment, where she is comfortable and clearly at home. All eight members of Donna's circle were at that meeting. We talked freely and openly about Donna's strengths, experience with children, and our plans to help Donna become a good mother to her child. The CAS worker ended the meeting by saying that no file would be opened on Donna, and if that other young mothers got the kind of support that Donna was now getting, there would be very few mothers on her caseload at all.

The Coordinator Cannot 'Hold' the Circle Indefinitely

In the event of a crisis, our model is that the coordinator will work with the family to 'hold' the circle. This may mean assist in calling the circle together, facilitate the work that the circle must do in order to get through the crisis (schedule support for awhile, work on a funding proposal, recruit Supporters, keep communication going, etc.), or providing some direct support. This is especially the case when the crisis is happening to the parent, rather than to the supported individual directly.

However, even with the luxury of a group the small size of ours, it is physically and mentally impossible for one part-time coordinator to hold this role for more than one person at a time. For this reason it is imperative that such situations be seen as short term crisis interventions alone.

Furthermore, it is not in the interest of our long term goals and dreams to rely so fully on a paid person over a long period of time. We need to work to develop and rely on the personal, committed relationships that we believe make the real difference in people's lives. When the coordinator slips from being a bridge to those kinds of relationships, to actually being the relationship, then we have slipped into a paid-for service world. This is not the one on which we believe we can rely.

Some Broader Thoughts on Relationship

Interpersonal relationships, built on trust and commitment, seem to be the human way of making it through life in meaningful ways. People vary in their tolerance for the number, intensity, variation and personal satisfaction with relationship, but they do not waver in their desire and need for relationship.

We know this is true for ourselves. We know that it is equally true for our family members who have a disability. In fact, our experiences have brought us to agree with those who understand that vulnerable people—those who live on the margins of society due to perceived weakness or differences—need personal committed relationships based on trust and commitments to safeguard their very lives. A friend of mine has a brother with a developmental disability who lives with his family in their family home. My friend says that over the years as she was growing up with her brother, she understood that the only thing between her brother and the institution door was people. In crisis after crisis, it is only people that make the difference.

Within the families of Deohaeko, we were certain about the importance of relationship in the lives of our family members. A constant eye and ear to the possibility of relationship dictates our work at all times.

At first, during the initial few years of helping our family members come to live at Rougemount and call it home, we were open, welcoming, and very hopeful for each person who came to share any kind of relationship with our sons and daughters. Within the co-operative, we found ways to help new neighbours get to know our sons and daughters and be comfortable in their presence. We were friendly and helpful to all those we encountered in the hallways, laundry and meeting rooms. We helped neighbours begin to understand that they might expect practical assistance from our sons and daughters and their Supporters. We were kind to new work colleagues, supportive and helpful to placement students, and generally sympathetic and often very helpful to new Supporters. Basically, we were nice people to have around, and given half a chance we found ways to turn attention to the similar qualities of our sons and daughters.

For the most part, however, we were reactive rather than proactive to the opportunities of relationship around us. We were grateful for the many lovely people who began to come into the lives of our family member. We did not spend a lot of time questioning from where they had come, and certainly not why. To us, it would seem like the grace of God determined the appearance of certain key people coming into our lives.

Over time, we have slowly become more proactive about this process. Possibly this is because we are getting older and feel a need to bring some greater influence upon this most vital area in the lives of our family members. Possibly because not enough people stayed and became true friends through the hit-and-miss approach of the first years. Possibly because we felt that we were missing out on personal commitment within the friendships that had begun.

We began to realize that there were things we could do to influence the likelihood of a relationship developing in the first place, and then helping friends move toward greater personal commitment. Chapter 7 is all about a way of thinking about and being proactive about relationship. Our thoughts are built on the premise that we cannot create relationship, but we can recognize, encourage, and design opportunities in which the miracle of relationship is more likely to occur. This thinking has had a great impact on how we help people spend their time, how we think about support, and how we view relationship.

A discussion with Cathy Bloomfield, who has been friends with Caroline Ann for over 13 years, helps to highlight the value of being intentional and thoughtful about supporting new and fledgling relationships. She understands that although she and Caroline Ann liked each other and enjoyed spending time together from the start, it was Caroline Ann's mother, Helen's nurturing of this relationship early on that has made it so strong today. "I needed this," reflected Cathy recently. "I was single and working full-time, with two young boys. I was too busy to initiate things, too extended to be able to accept invitations that did not include my boys. Helen made it easy. She just brought our two families together. It was a family thing, and over time, that meant that Caroline Ann became like a sister to me. We've grown up together in many ways, and our families are now interwoven. She has seen my sons grow up, and she is a friend, and a fan who loves and cares about not just me, but all of us."

From this time together—slowly and over time in ways that met Cathy's phase in her life—Cathy identifies the mutuality in their relationship. "I have a tendency to complicate things, and Caroline Ann does not. She has a way of showing me a more simple way, turning my burden into a freedom. When I am *really* with her, things in my day are pared to their essential. It is straight forward, no guessing. This is a pleasure and a freedom."

The second important thing we began to understand was that part of developing personal commitment between friends is to not have others think all is rosy and sunshine all of the time. As well as talking shared interests, shared spaces, and gifts, we need to talk to people about vulnerability. We need to offer them a role—not too overwhelming—a chance at being a part of a bigger whole. We began to realize that our own continual efforts to show how well we could manage would leave no obvious need or role for a personal commitment from others.

Finally, we began to truly see the personal relationships that were developing around us with very little intervention from ourselves. We began to see that while we were focused on age-peers to some extent, people were telling us they were also interested in intergenerational relationships.

Brenda and Hilda have met for tea most weekdays for almost ten years. It was Hilda who discovered and gently deepened Brenda's appreciation for listening to stories read aloud. And Hilda has always been clear on why the relationship works for them. "Brenda can walk away if she wants to when she's with me. If she doesn't want to come, she stays home. When she is ready to leave, she goes home."

David is five years old and lives at Rougemount. Part of almost every day includes time with his half-sister, Tiffany. Perhaps he just runs in to say "hi" before kindergarten. Or maybe he comes in the afternoon for awhile longer and offers to take Tiffany's shoes off for her. He knows that her feet need good circulation. He is intrigued by her *Glucoscan* which measures the sugar in her blood, and can already help with many parts of the procedure. He likes to sit and watch movies with Tiffany. Some days she and her mother walk him over to the library for new books. In the winter when his own mother was working a night shift, he stayed the night in Tiffany's apartment. He has spent a lot of time with Tiffany and will let others know when he thinks she is telling him something that needs to be done. He understands her well and is often right.

We also learn deeply from our ongoing struggles. Are all of our stories about relationship success stories? Of course not, and as with the rest of human endeavour, it is often within the failures that we learn our most important lessons. And in the midst of perceived failure, there are often intermingled moments of hope and promise.

Rob's Relationships

Rob's circle struggles endlessly with the challenges of moving from friendly welcomes and encounters into true relationship. For a long time, we saw him as well engaged with many people in his community, but without stronger ties to anyone. As our worry and frustration grew, we began to look harder. We started to see things in a different way.

Rob is a tall, quiet man who likes to be on the move in and around many places in his community. He loves to be around action and people, but by nature, he is an observer of people. He does not like to touch or hold things very much, and his communications are often so subtle that only those who have known him over time can catch his humour and his feelings for the situation. Rob has periods of intense seizure activity that require most people some time to feel comfortable around. These things have meant that finding strong, positive roles for Rob in his community has demanded much thought and creativity. Over time, Rob has come to be the owner of a very small courier company, *Rob's Small Parcel Delivery*. He is a member of a senior men's swim group, and a volunteer at his grandmother's nursing home providing quiet visits to people. He is a regular member of the library, and a regular fan of the Ajax Community Orchestra. On weekends he volunteers at a local wild animal sanctuary. As a co-operative member, Rob has some regular responsibilities delivering mail among his neighbours. He has become the main organizer (with considerable assistance) of the annual Rougemount camping trip. He is a long-time member of the Rosary Group in the co-operative. Every week, Rob is involved with all of the routine tasks of keeping his home in good shape—cleaning, shopping, banking, etc. On weekends, Rob spends a fair bit of his time with parents and visits together with his brothers and sister and their families. These roles have developed over time and have helped Rob shape a fairly full and busy routine most weeks—just the way he likes it.

On the face of it, Rob's life has led him into regular contact with many different people in many different settings in community. He is greeted warmly by many, many people wherever goes. Men from the swim club, staff from the nursing home, employees from the library, bank and grocery store, members of the orchestra, customers from his courier business, and many co-operative members find time and occasion to seek him out and speak with him a bit. However, deeper relationship seems to elude him.

We talked with each other, with Supporters, with neighbours and with other family members. Slowly, another picture began to emerge. We've noticed that Rob's Supporter, John, has been with Rob for about 9 years, and throughout that time Rob has had an emerging relationship with John's three young nephews, now well into their teens.

They camped and vacationed together almost every summer and winter. They boys have spent many hours with John at Rob's. Although, there is yet no independent relationship between any of the nephews and Rob, there is great personal knowledge and understanding. This story is not yet over.

We've remembered that Nihal, another Supporter of long standing, has told us about Rob's wonderful relationship with Susie that lasted two years. Susie was a friend of Nihal's, and a woman with a beautiful garden who made room for Rob—first in her garden by finding a small flower box that he could tend without bending down so far. Then she made room in her living room, by ensuring that Rob had a favourite chair to sit in whenever he came by, no matter how crowded the house might be. She made room for Rob in her family, by inviting him to partake in *Eid* celebrations one year. The ending of this relationship is a story and a lesson in itself, for it is linked to problems between Susie and the Supporter's family. It had nothing to do with Rob, except that he lost a new friend. We learned that this lovely relationship had not left the safe boundaries of the Supporter's presence. It had not yet had a chance to become an independent relationship between Rob and Susie. And then we were too late. Nonetheless, it was evidence of the possibility of that kind of relationship for Rob, and we take heart in that piece.

We've seen that Carol, who lives in the co-operative and who cuts Rob's hair, knows him well and finds ways to seek him out and make sure he is well. The Rosary Group often takes place at her home, and Rob has a special chair for himself there as well.

And finally, we are reminded that all of the many others who greet Rob warmly and kindly are a rich resource of potential relationship that we have yet to dip into.

What we have learned from Rob is that relationship building or inviting takes great care and attention.

Supporters spend a lot of time with Rob being present with the same people over and over again. They are engaged in a great balancing act. Initially, they must support Rob to be present and their support is vital. Later, they must step back and encourage the relationship to take hold for its own sake. This we have done less well, and will guide our efforts in the future. Perhaps most importantly, we all need to believe that personal relationship is possible for Rob, and that both parties will benefit from a deep relationship with this wonderful man.

I want to touch on the some of the outcomes of our work and focus on relationship. What difference has all of this made in the real lives of the sons and daughters of the Deohaeko families? It is all just fancy words if we cannot point to some real relationships that have brought life and enrichment to people. The relationships below have not come about solely because of circles in people's lives. However, we have used circles as a way to hold a vision of a good life, as a way to invite some people into the lives of individuals, and as a way to remind ourselves of the importance of relationship. Circles have helped us to make sure that people are leading lives where they are more inclined to meet people. Circles have reminded us all that these individuals are loving, interesting and worthy members of our community, in short, pretty decent folk to be holding up one end of a relationship.

This is a sampling of what this focus has brought to us:

Tiffany has had a warm and loving relationship with her five-year old half-brother, David, since birth. David lives at Rougemount and sees Tiffany daily. Sandi, once a roommate of Tiffany moved out six months ago, but their friendship is finding new ground. Sandi works nearby and finds ways to visit Tiffany almost every week. With the birth of her first niece, Britney, Tiffany is entering into a new relationship with her brother Joel and Lisa. Important friends at Rougemount include Janice, Gaytri, Lynn and others. Through her work in the Rouge Valley, Tiffany has warm collegial relations with several of the other environmental staff and volunteers.

Brenda continues to share tea most days at 4:00 with her dear friend and next-door neighbour, Hilda. Although she usually avoids young children, Brenda has developed a great fondness for Matthew, Donna's son and buys him treats and small gifts often. Brenda has a great working relationship with the man, Dave Ryan, who helped her get to council to petition for her park site. She does not see him often, but he looks out for her at the annual Volunteer Awards Dinner. He has also recently become mayor of Pickering, so Brenda knows some people in high places. Brenda has a quiet friendship with Gaytri who lives at Rougemount and a number of neighbours who come to her rescue at various times. She has become closer to her sister-in-law, Barb, and brother Martin over the past year.

Jon had a wonderful working relationship with the police sergeant at a local station where he had a shredding contract for several years. He has great work relationships with several of his shredding customers. He has a special relationship with Carol, who used to support him, and her whole family. They all live in the building. He continues to spend time with a family in Uxbridge. As always, he loves his time with his sister Rebecca, his aunt Maureen and his Aunt Brenda, and his Gran.

Rob has a good relationship with his neighbour Carol, with Hilda, as well as with several other neighbours. He travels frequently with his Supporter John and his nephews. Rob has work-related friends that he encounters through his volunteer work at the nursing home, wildlife park, and his courier business. He has forged good recreational links with people through his interest in the local orchestra and his swimming club. Several people have become friends and then have moved out of his life again—a bittersweet experience to be sure.

John has a close and wonderful friendship with George who is the chef of the nearby restaurant. He has a good working relationship with Kim, Stella and many other of the wait staff there. John has a longstanding hockey friendship with an elderly neighbour, Art, from an old neighbourhood. He also is still busily spending time with the many members of Jeany's family.

Caroline Ann has a long and close friendship with Cathy, whom she has known for many years. She keeps in touch with Nicola, the principal of the Montessori school across the street from the co-operative and stops in whenever she is at Rougemount. Theresa and Donna are two close friends for her at the co-operative, and she keeps in touch with Kim from the nearby restaurant. Several close and important friendships have changed quickly and painfully for Caroline Ann over the past two years. These are difficult blows to overcome. Her nephew Terry has brought very special dimensions to her life, especially since she has always shared a warm relationship with her sister, Barb.

As outlined above, Donna has a wide and elaborate circle of friends. She also has good neighbours in Susanna and her family. The depth and breadth of Donna's circle is a testament to the priority she places on people in her life.

And from where do these relationships come? The answer to this question is an important one, and one that we will come back to several times in later chapters. For now, let us understand that the deepest relationships described above have come about through family connections (sisters and brothers having children, nieces and nephews growing up and seeing this aunt or uncle in a new way), determined personal efforts of single circle members, parents recognizing and personally encouraging new friendships, and regular, intense presence in familiar community settings (within Rougemount, at a nearby restaurant) day after day after day. One or two connections may be directly attributed to a keen, creative Supporter, but the majority stem from family, from long-time friends, and from the individual's own personal attractions once they are assisted to be in the same valued setting on a regular basis holding a familiar and valued role.

A strong sense of home is like a taproot for people's lives and we have seen in the previous chapter that this root runs deep and secure for the people of Deohaeko. The roots of relationship as explored in this chapter are then the side roots. They provide for stability and growth, offering their many or fewer numbers to prevent lives from falling over or becoming uprooted. The next chapter will look to what a widening sense of community spaces offers to people's lives.

Chapter 5
A Greater Sense of Place

From the insights and successes gained from 'home' as the first sense of place, people have gathered the confidence to begin to look outward to other parts of the community with greater interest.

Our community is a wide and varied place. For us, it includes a co-operative community where opportunities range from mandatory General Members Meetings to committee meetings to community potlucks, the Rosary group, clean up events and spontaneous get-togethers. It includes a community of relationships involving a growing number of close and extended family members, friends, co-workers, church and club members and more. It is also a geographical community of the local business community comprised of the restaurants, banks, the library, the local community garden, shops, hair dressers, fitness studio, convenience stores, doctors and dentists all within walking distance of the co-operative. Farther out it includes the greater community of interests where people travel greater distances to link to places of work, civic, or leisure-related interests.

This is our community—a sense of place that is intertwined with identity and belonging. But first, we had to learn to see it and that is a story in itself.

There are two important assumptions—points of principle—that we have always made that must be addressed before we go further: One, people do not have to be 'ready' to enter this part of their lives, and two, people do not come and go in and out of community.

'Ready' for Community

We do not think about people in terms of being 'ready' for their roles in community. We did not have a period of focusing on 'home' and 'people who care' and then when that came to an end, that we moved on to helping people to look out and figure their roles and places within the greater community. This would imply that people had to get ready inwardly in some way before venturing out into their community. That is not at all what happened here. People did not have to be ready in order to begin to live their lives outside of their front door. This all happened at the same time. They were simply living more and more full lives. As they became more clear on what home meant for them and we became more clear on supporting them in those very ways, our efforts—which had been going on from the beginning and had never stopped—to find and enter into meaningful roles in community seemed to become more effective and satisfying.

In part, we had been working very hard at listening to and understanding what people wanted, and doubtlessly our enhanced skills in these areas were brought into play here, too. We were better at figuring out what people were telling us and wanting us to understand.

In part, we had been together for quite awhile by this time, and so had more experience at assessing and judging the quality and potential of different opportunities. We were probably gaining skills and more able to make things work than we had been before.

But all of that aside, there was also some measure of things working out in community roles and participation that could be more directly attributed to people's growing sense of personal space. They were beginning to more clearly understand who they were and what they had to offer to their community. They were emotionally and psychologically, perhaps, more prepared to enter into expanding and enriching this part of their lives.

'In Community'

Just as there is no prerequisite of 'getting ready' to move into community connections and roles in our model, there is also no sense of spending some time 'in the community'. When people live in typical arrangements right within a typical community, there is no sense of 'moving into the community' or going into the community for any part of one's day or week. They are always in community, part of the community. They are community.

This has been a revolutionizing concept that our language does not even prepare us for. We often talk about going into the community as if it were another place. For you or I—typical citizens—this is just the way we talk. Our lives are so full of potential and demands that we mean that we intentionally move into greater or lesser contact with the members of our community. Of course, we do not physically move in or out of any real community space, but we speak in this shorthand, among ourselves who understand fully the reality we live. Of key significance is the fact that we are in full control of the degree and time to which we are in greater or lesser contact with other members of our community.

People who have been shunned and segregated from typical community life have truly experienced being 'in community' one moment, and then being well and truly 'out of the community' the next. They have had their lives scheduled in such a way that some parts of their day are deliberate attempts to have them spend time among typical members of the community. They have little say or control over how much time and what kind of contact they may enter into with other members of that community.

The individuals within Deohaeko, however, live in their own apartment homes where they have had much say over where the apartment is, how it is decorated, who (else) lives there, who visits, and what they do within their homes. They also spend most of their time with a close family member, friend, or well-oriented one-to-one Supporter. Each of these individuals knows the person very well and attempts within a broader framework to design their day, week, general life to suit their goals, dreams, and day-to-day moods.

Therefore, to a degree that has not been previously afforded to most individuals with an intellectual disability, the people who are supported through Deohaeko truly are in community. To celebrate this victory, and in order to not lose consciousness about its importance, we try very much not to speak the language of 'in and out of community'.

We do not speak about people 'going into the community' today. We do not plan for a person's daytime hours as if she were attending a day program that was focused on the community. We do not separate what people do in the daytime from what they do in the evenings—we try to support people wherever and whenever support needs to happen in order for the person to be doing and being what they desire most. We make sure that many roles that the person holds are supported by unpaid family members and friends. It is not a program, it is life.

This is our community, then, that combination of co-operative community, relationships, local geographic community and broader community of interests. All of it is a sense of place intertwined with identity and belonging. But we had to learn to see it, and that is an important part of this story.

We needed to re-discover the community and its potential that lay at our doorstep. To do so, we had, first of all, to understand the stresses and complexities of our current society that hide true community from our quick glance. Then, we had to re-discover our part in recognizing and encouraging the remnants of hospitality in our midst. Finally, armed with our new knowledge, we had to be able to design new and effective opportunities to be involved in true community. Once again, our path to learning and understanding is only clear and simple in retrospect. In fact, we were clear about our role in recognizing and encouraging hospitality right from the start. Our initial understanding of intentional community had fostered this within us. But our efforts became more effective once we better understood the hostility of much of current society to vestiges of true welcome and community. And even today, it is often when our efforts at implementation are stymied that we look back and realize where we have fallen off the path again. The way is rocky and often uncertain, but some of the rest stops along the way are an oasis of hope and joy.

A part of the story of coming to see community as we do now, was my own opportunity to be away for a period of time in Holland in 2000. The time away with time for reading and reflection, and my subsequent return with the opportunity to look at this community with 'new eyes' was very helpful to thinking about our work.

A Tale of Two Cities

I went away with my family to Europe for three months during the summer of 2000. When I returned to Pickering, I was amazed and dismayed that the long stretch of city roadway between the co-operative and the small Tim Hortons coffee shop to the east had been totally re-developed. Before, between the co-operative and the next major intersection some 2 km to the east, on the co-operative side of the road, there had been a church, a stretch of ravine and green and undeveloped, neglected lots, and then a small food and department store, a plant nursery, the Tim Hortons and the corner gas station. Not a wildly exciting stretch of city road but it allowed the co-operative and its two small adjacent plazas a sense of being set a bit apart in its own neighbourhood. In addition, the Tim Hortons was one of the last of its kind—kind of old, a bit out-dated, and complete with the swivel stools lined up at the counter. The employees there tended to be older, or maybe just chattier, and no drive-thru existed at all. You lined up body-to-body with everyone else for your coffee and most mornings there was a long, chatty line of other coffee drinkers.

A few months later, that stretch of roadway had undergone a major transformation. Work was not yet complete but the plan was clear to see. A whole new plaza had sprung up with a huge parking lot. The Second Cup coffee shop, complete with drive-thru service, was in the new plaza, along with a large grocery chain store, a gigantic video rental franchise, (*check what else is there!*) At the far east corner of the plaza sat a fat new and gleaming Burger King...complete with drive-thru service.

The first thought that struck me was that there was no friendly-looking place to go in that square, white, new gleaming plaza. No sense of character except 'new and big' greeted my eyes. Clearly this was a place to drive to, not to walk to. People were to come from far away to use these stores. Even the parking lot attested to the fact that it was to entice many shoppers from many parts of the city to its stores. So even if you came here regularly, who would you know?

Secondly, I noticed three new traffic lights, two of them just to handle the flow of traffic into the new plaza areas. It felt so much busier—but in a car-not-people kind of way. I also saw a new sidewalk but the rush of the traffic along the road would make it smelly and unpleasant, and a place to walk only if you were forced to rather than for a stroll for your neighbourhood shopping. In fact, this stretch of roadway, although within the city limits of Pickering, has had a long standing problem with fast traffic. It used to be the old main highway and so it still feels to many drivers who like to gun it along that straight stretch. Now the three traffic lights check their pace a bit, but really serve only to frustrate them as they attempt to gun it along shorter and shorter distances. The walk to the friendly Tim Hortons would be less calming, that was for sure.

I did not feel drawn to any of the stores in the new plaza areas. They all looked big and bright and their signs proclaimed exactly what they were. There was no place for a curiosity shop of any kind—no store that showed any mystery and enticement to come and see its lure. I remember sighing, this was a big new aspect of my community where I needed to do 'my work'. I had been reading David Schwartz's book *Who Cares?* during my time in Holland and felt immediately that there would be few, if any, vestiges of true community in this bit of Pickering.

Part of what I felt was truly culture shock. I had spent three months in a small city in Holland's southernmost province of Limburg. My living experience had been very, very different. In Holland, by law, cities are limited to a certain size. They are permitted to take up only a certain amount of geographical space. When that is filled, they must build inward or else use up space in another city's allotment. As harsh as this appears, some wonderful things happen as a result of these practices. For one, because Holland is so densely populated (15 million people—half the number of Canadians—in a 41,000 square kilometre space the size of Vancouver Island) houses are typically small and efficient and small cities are still very full of people.

In Venray, for example, there live about 50,000 people. The city is of a size where a healthy adult can walk or bike easily to any part of the city. There are bike paths throughout the city—not just a line on the main thoroughfares, but actual paths separated by grassy boulevards to allow for the safe and efficient use of bike travel, even by very young, beginning, or unsteady bike riders. This being the case, you also see a wide range of accommodations in bike equipment. Motorized scooters and bikes accommodate those who have less energy for vigorous cycling. Three-wheeled versions assist many people who have difficulty with balance or coordination. These often come equipped with such vast basket and carrying areas, that they seem more practical for daily use than many of the streamlined versions. Separate, safe biking areas also mean less of a need for a bike helmet law and so virtually all except the youngest bikers enjoy helmet-free biking in their city.

Therefore it is not surprising that people bike everywhere. People bike to work in business suits and tight skirts, children bike to school from the youngest age to the oldest teens. People shop for all of their groceries on their bikes and have developed many ingenious bags and attachments to help carry heavy or awkward loads. People bike to the library, to town to run errands, to visit friends. Mothers and fathers can be seen carrying up to three children on one bike—one up front, and two in the back—all on approved seating arrangements. On evenings and weekends families bike together for fun and visiting. In the time that we were in Venray, we biked daily for all of our needs, although we had access to a car. I noticed that unless our tasks took us more than 15 km away, we would not even question whether to bike or to drive. Our son, at age eight then, had an odometer on his bike and clocked over 800 km in a 10-week period! Our four-year old daughter learned to bike in Holland and clocked 200 km of her own in addition to the hundreds of kilometres clocked on the back of my bike.

I go on at some lengths about this bike thing because it was central to daily life, and came about in part as a direct result of the size of the city. It also remains for me a very pleasant memory because of some of the other things that naturally happened because we were on a bike rather than in a car. First of all, we greeted everyone we met—substantial numbers in a day!—and the children could get by with their minimal Dutch quite fluently. We also had many small conversations at rest stops with other bikers, when we were locking up our bikes in the town, and many other places. We were simply more often face to face with others, and it felt rude not to talk. And so we became accustomed to making small talk with a wide variety of people. Secondly, we often stopped for a few minutes whenever we passed a playground. This just never came up in Canada when we pass playgrounds while driving around in a car. But for the children on a bike, the playground was so immediate and accessible (no need to find parking, for one!) that it was natural to stop. And of course, we made many other casual acquaintances in that way. Thirdly, we came to know our city in a very intimate way. We tried many different streets and paths, got lost and found our way again and again. By the end of three months we knew many of the best nooks and crannies of Venray, and showed them to other people. Not much in the way of new construction, changes in park areas, or passing fairs could easily pass us by.

So, in very concrete ways, city size encouraged continued bike use (already a cultural routine) which encouraged greeting and small talk among citizens and also encouraged our knowing our community in a very intimate way.

The other thing about Venray, despite its size and perhaps due to its dense population, is that it has practically every kind of shop or service that you could possibly want. There is really no reason to be going to any of the larger cities. One day we took a train to the border town of Venlo, and although it was fun to explore a new city, it had nothing in terms of shops, restaurants, specialities, churches or services that I had not already seen in Venray. Venray has a real city centre with a small, vibrant pedestrian zone where many shops compete for customers. There are a few chain stores, but even these are small due to the premium on space in the city. Every Monday is market day in the city and farmers who are literally located just on the edge of town, bring their truly fresh produce in for sale. This makes market days a festive occasion every week in Venray. There is a wide array of restaurants—sit down, take out, bistro, pub, etc. There are also a number of shops that specialize in food to be taken home all prepared for the supper table. The result is that although you can travel for many other reasons, you rarely do so just for shopping or to eat out. Travel is reserved for vacation, visiting, or events outside of the city.

I have gone into such detail about my Dutch living experience because the return to home in Canada, and to Pickering, in particular, was such a contrast. I hasten to say that I have drawn out of my Dutch experience a few aspects of life that make imminent sense to me and which shaped me for my particular reaction to returning to life in a small Canadian city. Dutch society has many struggles and challenges of its own, and many others which are very similar to ours. Despite some of the structural advantages that I have outlined above, even small cities like Venray are vulnerable to the ravages of the market economy on their ability to care for each other.

That being said, my own return to Pickering took some deep thinking.

Rediscovering Pickering

David Schwartz's book, *Who Cares?*, was very helpful in analyzing my experiences in these two cities. His analysis of the stresses of our current market-driven society and its impact on our communities was also helpful in coming to understand Pickering in new and impactful ways. He has written with wonderful clarity about an almost forgotten culture of hospitality within our neighbourhoods. He calls this diminishing culture which is tolerant, caring and creative the *vernacular* culture. People look after each other without being told or orchestrated and do so in small, local ways. This way of being there for one another amid the growing pressures of everyday life is rapidly disappearing.

And yet this is an essential culture for us to preserve and promote for it is within the vernacular culture that the people at the margins of fast-moving society are included and can gain a foothold. It is here that we can find hope for us all.

One of the most useful things that Schwartz enabled me to see was to learn to recognize places within our communities where vernacular culture was still likely to be found. And so I turned my back on the shiny, new and franchised elements of Pickering society and looked again.

I looked for the small, the family-owned, the local, the unhurried, the unique and the unconventional.

One of the first things that I was able to see was that the two plazas next door were more than ordinary strip malls. When I looked carefully I saw that they contained many of the small shops that are often displaced by full-service grocery stores in many areas. It turned out that they included a milk store, a butcher shop, a fruit and vegetable market, two convenience stores, four places to eat, a bank and a bank machine, a second hand children's clothing store, two places to get a haircut, an aerobics studio, a massage and physiotherapy office, and a pet supply shop. I saw how fully people were able to live in this walking community, and how people's lack of access to transportation fed into this loop wonderfully well. For most day-to-day errands and needs, people are well able to use these local shops and services. Most people and their families talk about shop keepers and small business owners in those two plazas by name and with personal detail. Shopkeepers and restaurant owners greet many of us by name, and ask a personal question or two that lets you know they are familiar with some aspects of your life.

And then, together with the families, I have been able to re-discover much richness, diversity and welcome within our Pickering area community. People have found welcome, acceptance and a true sense of place within those vestiges of vernacular culture in the Pickering area. We see two of the local restaurants with new eyes. We know the owners and the staff, and they know and welcome us. They know and welcome many of the Rougemount members, and have come to make subtle adaptations to their welcome as individual circumstances arise. The restaurant called *Kathryn's* welcomes John in unique ways and has created opportunity for a real friendship to grow between John and chef, George.

This also means that the local hairdresser knows Brenda well, and can gauge Brenda's patience in order to do a good job in a short time. The people at the dollar store know and expect Jon to arrive at the very beginning of each new holiday season as he begins to decorate his apartment. Tiffany is able to deal with the same person at the bank most times, and the milk store knows its ice-cream-lovers well.

We see that the *Ajax Community Orchestra* welcomes Rob as a regular to their weekly practices and members show their appreciation for his audience by including him at coffee time, and playing their various instruments for him as a private audience. The local wildlife sanctuary welcomes Brenda's visits and accepts Jon's shredded paper offerings from his own small business. The Montessori school across the street has welcomed and adapted to Caroline Ann's particular skills in ways that a larger school system would be unlikely to do. Brenda spends time at her park site because a local watershed rehabilitation project understood her need for place and created a new way to volunteer within their project. Donna is finding welcome at a local church down the road that her family had attended years ago. Tiffany has found purpose, welcome, and friendship among the volunteers and staff at the Rouge Valley Naturalists at their Pearse House space. Jon has discovered a number of welcoming places that give him space to work at his shredding contracts: a local police station, a high school office, a large corporation's office space, a dentist's office.

These community places of welcome had always been there. We have just learned so see them, to develop their potential, and to use them well. And the people that we support have told us clearly that it is important to have a few places outside of home, outside of Rougemount, where they belong, where they feel they can make a contribution, and where they are defined by others by what they can do rather than by what they cannot do.

Over the years, I have come to look at and for community in new ways. I am less deterred by rows of box malls and franchise restaurants because I have come to trust other ways of finding the vernacular community than simply looking up and down the street.

Look at public notices. I read community in much of the public information that floats about us. I read local newspapers, starting with the notices, advertisements, and back pages first. These are the places that tell me about what kinds of things people in this community are interested in. I am not just looking for what people are invited to do as 'participants', but also what kinds of organizing, planning and coordinating role people are taking on. I read library bulletin boards, recreation centre schedules (especially the back sections), and bulletin boards of all kinds. Our world is full of written information about what ordinary people are doing with their time. Many of them are keen to connect with others who share their interests or who are just curious to know more about their passion.

Find out more about the people you already know. Through our circle gatherings, and especially the larger brainstorming gatherings that we have tried out for a number of people, we discover that many people whom we know in one kind of way, have a host of interests and skills that link them to many different places in the community. This also helps to fill in my sense of what other 'unseen' places and gatherings of people make up this community.

Jon's shredding business really got moving when we were able to figure out what kinds of people required shredding, and then realizing we already knew some people like that. Most of Jon's business has not come about through advertising or cold calls, but through personal links by people who know him well.

Walk instead of drive. I find it helpful to slow down and actually walk through an area in the community and try to figure out what takes place in its nooks and crannies. I was quite surprised at one time when I tried to map out the two local plazas near Rougemount. I did the best I could and then walked over to check my map against reality. I had forgotten about one third of the businesses, shops and services offered in the little plazas. Most of these were not immediately useful to me but I filed them away in my mind for future reference. Also, when walking, it is possible to see and read signage that is not seen from a car. I have learned to ask myself what these mean and what the people in these places might be doing.

John's Sense of Place

John's story reminds me to listen to the stories happening around me in order to find the community under my nose.

John is a quiet man who warms up to people on his own terms. He is a night owl who loves sports, especially the Toronto Maple Leafs, his local team the Oshawa Generals, and in summer, the Montreal *Expos*. John reads the paper for statistics, standings and game schedules. There is not much about these sports that John does not know. He tends to move around the co-operative quietly, not talking to his neighbours unless he feels very comfortable with them. When John started living on his own his father was a bit worried about John feeling lonely, without easy access to people he would want to see. Doug did not think that John would easily knock on a neighbour's

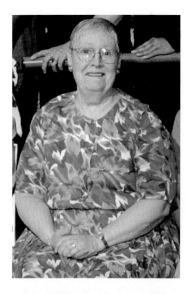

Marje Mitchell (1931 – 2003)

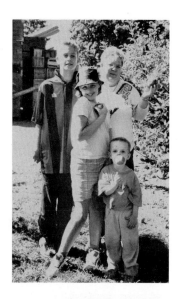

Donna and Matthew Mitchell
with friends at the
apple orchard.

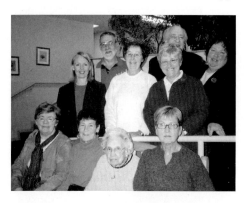

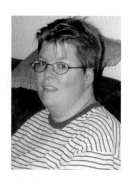

Front Row	Linda Dawe, Elizabeth Gray, Hilda Hawkes, Mary Bennett	Donna
Middle Row	Janet Klees, Harriet Salmers Helen Dionne	
Back Row	Doug Hobson, Orest Salmers, Janice Salsbury	
Absent	Clive Bennett, George Dionne, Margaret Presutti	

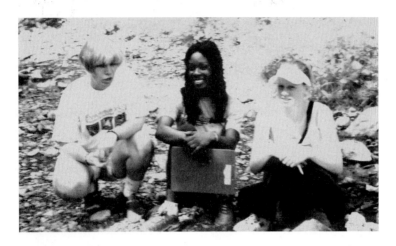

Brenda Gray (far left) as an environmental steward at her park site with co-workers.

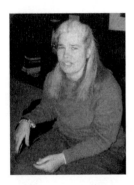

Brenda

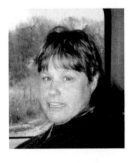

Caroline Ann

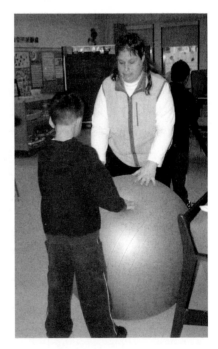

Caroline Ann Dionne, teaching assistant at the local school.

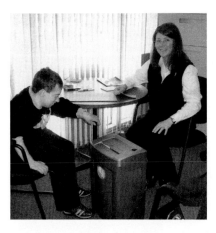

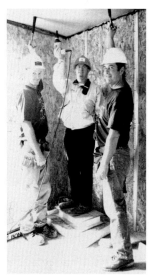

Jon Bennett, owner of *J.B. Shredding,* with a customer.

John Hobson (centre) HABITAT FOR HUMANITY volunteer with two fellow volunteers.

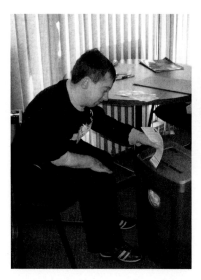

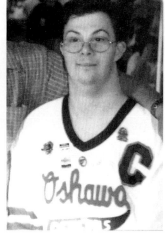

Jon

John

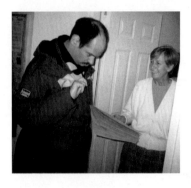

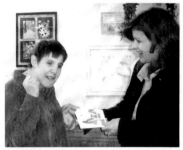

Rob Salmers, courier, on a
delivery to a local organization

Tiffany Dawe (left) discussing
her art cards with *Green Thumb*
shop owner, Shelley.

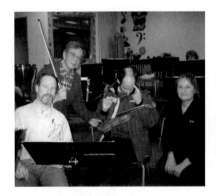

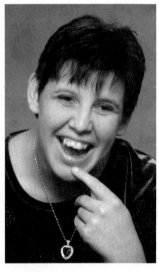

Rob and members of the Ajax
Community Orchestra

Tiffany

door for a visit. He also hoped to find some other young people that John could hang around.

The people in John's small circle started to think about this, as well as our ongoing concern about the lack of a stable job for John. He had a lot of free time in his day and we began to take notice of where he went and what he did with his time.

We noticed that he would go to the restaurant in the plaza next door nearly every day for coffee, and on Thursdays for supper. *Kathryn's Fish and Chip Restaurant* is well known for its great breakfasts, fish and chips and televising of evening sports. We noticed that although the owners were of Doug's generation, the chef (who was the owners' son) and the rest of the staff were all younger people closer to John's age. We saw that John was greeted warmly by the staff, and more importantly, that he spoke to them in return. George, the chef and another cook also share John's love of sports and traded statistics and opinions of the previous night's games. We decided that we would see about solidifying John's already positive presence in the restaurant.

With John's agreement, I spoke with the owners about John coming on Tuesday nights to help close down the restaurant. We chose this time because it would not be overly busy with customers but there would be a number of routine tasks to be done (sweeping, putting up chairs) that John could do. It would be late at night, which not only suited John's preference for staying up late, but also meant that the staff would be all working together as a team. Mary and Tony, the owners, looked surprised at the request, but agreed that John could help out in this way.

John clearly knew most of the staff and also knew a fair bit about restaurant work from previous experience, so we decided that having someone turn up with him for support would be unnecessary and intrusive. Instead, Doug called him on Tuesdays to remind him of his commitment, and then checked out with him how it was going. Doug also popped in on Tuesday nights every few weeks to make sure that things looked and felt good. I frequently use the restaurant for interviews and small meetings, and would casually ask Mary or George from time to time how things were going.

John worked hard and his work was appreciated. He worked with four or five young people who bantered easily among themselves, including John in their chatter. George seemed to take the lead on directing John to chores that needed to be done. Over the next while, we watched many positive developments. John began to drop by the restaurant most nights of the week. George said they could count on him to arrive after the second period of a hockey game, or after the seventh inning of a baseball game. He argued with the staff and a few patrons about the game, took control of the television remote for the evening and stayed to help out with a few chores. After awhile, he started coming by on the weekends before or after spending time with his family. He was soon invited to pull himself drinks from the soda fountain whenever he wanted. I have seen him take on many different jobs over the years. John celebrates his birthday and Christmas with the staff every year. George calls him to check up on him when he doesn't come in as expected just to make sure that he is alright. John has gone out with Chris, the dishwasher to hear his band play.

Not too long after this, John found a position at a local Burger King for a few hours every day. This was a paid position and he likes earning money. We were not sure what would happen with Kathryn's but we trusted John to figure things out. He did. He goes into Kathryn's after work in the afternoons most days. It's a place to talk to people about his day and unwind with a coffee. Lately, with the server Kim's assistance he has also started to serve coffee to some of the tables. This is another achievement for a shy guy who has not liked to greet people he does not know.

He returns most evenings to help close the restaurant, and he still is there on the weekend. It's clear that John does not feel pressured to be there, but chooses to spend his time at a place that knows and welcomes him. He feels appreciated and needed. He has a place where he can talk to friends and co-workers when he chooses.

Several times over the past years, we have talked about pay for John. So far, each time we have decided against asking for pay for some of the following reasons. John comes and goes at the restaurant as he pleases. He certainly helps out in ways that make a difference and in some ways, people count on him as well. He likes this feeling, but he feels that he is an equal to all of the people in the restaurant. He is giving something of himself that he alone controls. We think that pay would be linked to certain hours and certain expectations. Would he feel that he could not come in at the other times. Would people begin to supervise him or direct him differently? These are not chances that we feel prepared to take right now. John has found his 'third' place, as David Schwartz calls it—a place of community right around the corner from his home.

Last year, Mary and Tony sold their restaurant. We waited with bated breath to meet the new owners. Although I went to the restaurant the minute I heard the news, the new owners had been there for three days already. My first sign of relief was to see George cooking behind the grill. I then met Stella, the new owner, as she served me my coffee. I casually asked how John was doing, and she sat down and enthusiastically told me that he was just fine and everyone just loved him there! I also talked to George about his plans and he said that he would be staying on for awhile, and when he did leave John would always know where to find him. Things looked promising, but still we worried about the future. After several weeks of watching and waiting (two imminently useful and not valued enough strategies for community building), I had a conversation with Stella. Her initial understanding of John's place, role and importance within Kathryn's has been heartening. The waiting and watching had paid off well, since John's own presence, charm and dedication to the restaurant and its staff had proved his worth in a way that my few words or interference could never have done.

Doing Our Part: Supporting a Culture of Hospitality

David Schwartz outlines six useful actions that people can take to support this culture of hospitality in which we all thrive more fully. In many ways, the work that the families of Deohaeko have undertaken over the years can be understood and even strengthened by drawing parallels with David Schwartz's six actions.

The first action involves *slowing down the destruction of the vernacular culture*—being aware of how the powers of a market economy cannot operate hand in hand with hospitality, but in fact, must weed out vestiges of hospitality in order to stay their course. The mainstays of hospitality—small, unique gestures that are often slow, imperfect and able to take many exceptions into account and may have different answers to the same problem— cannot be present in a thriving market economy. The first action is then, one of *awareness* and taking action to follows this cardinal rule: *no social activity permitted that destroys a current practice that is small, local and able to accommodate people in unique responsive ways.*

The building of Rougemount and its intentional community is a clear example, with many smaller stories within, of our work in this regard. A few elderly people living at Rougemount have been helped to continue to live in their homes with the help of neighbours and family, far beyond what is typical in other parts of the community where they might be seen as best served in a nursing home. Rougemount's mantra of being good neighbours to one another is a good way of making sure that the first level of assistance is simply a helping hand from a neighbour. In fact, we have been careful never to establish a public and obvious office for Deohaeko within the Rougemount community. We felt that by not doing so, we could be more sure that if help is needed by one of the members of Deohaeko, turning to a neighbour would be the first option. Then, calling the emergency in-house service would be the second option open to all members, and then for us, calling on the family would be the third option. All of these are typical, familiar routes for all co-operative members.

In small, local ways the sons and daughters of Deohaeko families are able to participate, give of themselves and be a part of a vibrant mutuality rather than the receiver of charity.

It is under this first action of being aware of and upholding that which is able to welcome people in unique ways, that I place my thoughts about the work that many colleagues, families, and others engage in currently in order to build and strengthen community and individual connections.

For the most part, I have noticed that we often approach the community and our hopes for the potential it may yield, in a typically Canadian way. We regard community as an endless renewable resource which is ours to exploit and plunder, and we spend little time worrying about the collateral damage that might arise when a connection does not work out, or a relationship does not thrive. At most, we worry about what the failed connection might mean for the person that we support. Rarely, do we take time to dwell on what this experience might mean for the other parties involved. We act as if this resource of community is rich and endless, and we can simply move on to new areas. As Canadians, we do the same with our minerals, our forests, and our water—discover, exploit, plunder, and move on. In some ways, it seems that community development-minded people do the same thing with the richness of community resources.

In part, this attitude comes from the professionalizing of community space and turning it into a commodity. We seem to regard community as an entity separate from ourselves and our lives, rather than as a living, breathing organism into which we—all of us—are integrally woven. Many people approach their time and connecting as 'work' and what we do with it remains quite separate from what we do with the rest of our lives. We meet people, ask for opportunities, introduce new people, and encourage relationships. But we often do this separately from the living that we do in other spaces of our home community.

This separateness allows us to view the connecting and relationship building as something that happens 'over there'. It is not a far leap to move from this kind of thinking to viewing community resources as a commodity that can be exploited (even for the best of the intentions). This means that we waste opportunities, people, and the energy within the community. We do not borrow and gently use. We plunder, use up and cast aside opportunities that do not seem perfect at first hand.

The collateral damage that results from this approach to our work is significant, but all too often we ignore it. In our exploitative approach to developing community, we often do not take the time to make things right with a failed connection before moving on to a better match. We do not take the time to thank people for the opportunities afforded (including the rich lessons that come to us through failure), the time that they have spent, or the efforts they have made. We do not help people realize that the match that did not work is an occasion for learning and moving forward, and not for blaming and feeling inadequate. We do not leave people with words that allow them to remain open and welcoming to another opportunity in the future with someone else who may be a better match.

Instead, when things go wrong or don't move at all, we usually abandon the potential connection with little thought or effort toward the people involved in that situation. Sometimes, we do not return at all, we simply end with an abrupt phone call, or we simply come less and less often until our final absence is hardly missed. Ironically, we often, thus, cast into stone the very images and vulnerabilities that we wish to avoid. The individual person with a disability remains little known to the people involved in the community situation, and therefore, their lasting impression is added to the growing perception that 'people with disabilities' are different, don't belong, can't commit, really have nothing to contribute, and are unreliable.

Over the years, as this attitude and approach to building involvement in community has become more clear to me, I have tried to model and encourage a different way in all of my endeavours to work within our communities. For one, I try to understand that I am a part of the community that I am seeking to build. In this way, the community is not other for the most part, it is *of me*. I do not want to act in exploitive ways any more than I, myself, would wish to be exploited. Two, I am compelled to act in gentle, respectful ways that seek to work toward the long term health and strength of the whole community—for the benefit of the person I support, for the benefit of this new person in our community, and for my own benefit and that of my family. Three, I am aware that the opportunities that might best sustain and welcome a person with a disability are those within the vernacular culture, as defined by David Schwartz.

These decisions mean that I understand the situations that could best welcome and accommodate a person with a disability are currently at risk of disappearing within our society. The opportunities that I discover, therefore, are rare, limited, and should be approached with great care and respect. If the opportunity does not lead to the connection that I had hoped, then I should leave it intact for the next person to try. Practically speaking, these thoughts lead me to do my work in the following ways.

I try to both start and end opportunities and connections respectfully. I try to share my experiences, lessons, joy and respect for relationship in all opportunities of which I become a part. I try to ensure that any one place in community is not overwhelmed with getting to know and welcome too many people with a disability. I try to become better and better at making a good match which includes benefiting both parties in the relationship (working, leisure, or otherwise). I try to be conscious of how my paid role in community might do irreparable damage to the goodwill of ordinary citizens and restrain myself from taking those actions. I make sure that I take off my paid coordinator hat regularly, and move into a personal, welcoming role in relationships with vulnerable people around me.

This approach takes a bit longer, but I believe it is another small, significant way to recognize people as individuals, to respect the struggle of all citizens for belonging and welcome, and to support a healthy, sustaining path for the kind of community in which I would like to live.

The second action is to *promote connecting of strangers who are unlikely to meet*. This involves people taking on the task of asking: asking people to meet, asking on behalf of people, and recognizing when there is a question to be asked that will improve the lot of both parties. This is based on the belief that enough hospitable culture remains that it can be stimulated by someone taking on the role of asker.

Within Deohaeko, at different times, families, Supporters or I take on this asking role. We ask for ways that people can volunteer, work, contribute and participate so that the final outcome enriches both the individual whose presence is offered, and the individual who finds a way to welcome. We make sure that we connect people who have a skill that fits the situation, a shared interest to pursue, or a particular presence to offer. Connecting people is one of the basic foundations of our work. Later on in this book (Chapters 6 and 7) we will discuss in detail all of the thought and intent that we put into this aspect of our work.

The third action is to ***stimulate associational groups*** by joining them and adding to their strength while extending your own personal network at the same time. These groups bring sometimes unlikely people to work on a common enterprise outside of the group. All members are stretched to work at new things in order to advance the work of the group. The focus is on the work at hand—the common passion—rather than the similarities or differences of the group members.

The people we support have joined and continue to strengthen a rich diversity of associational groups in the Pickering area. These include an art guild, a naturalist's group, several churches, a community orchestra, a rosary group, a swim club, an environmental project, a cultural association and many more. Often their presence has resulted in some alteration of how things are typically done, some adjustment by key members to ensure welcome, and some time to establish comfort and familiarity. On the other hand, the new members often show considerable efforts to be reliable and contributing participants. This together with time has almost always led to satisfying experiences all around.

Tiffany has always loved Irish and Celtic music, and when a new Irish Club was established in Pickering, she was eager to become involved. We called the information number, found out about the Open House, and helped Tiffany attend an evening of her favourite music and dance. We felt welcome—Irish or not—and Tiffany joined as a new member that night. Now she receives their regular newsletter of events, and invites friends and co-operative members to join her in attending. She has become familiar to the new group, and is currently organizing with some of them to play for her next birthday party. This latest event has a wonderful mutual quality to it as it allows Tiffany to enjoy an evening of music and friends, it offers her friends an evening together with entertainment, and it offers the Irish musicians a chance to increase their audience.

The fourth action is to recognize and **champion 'third places'.** These are the neighbourhood places that are small, local and independently owned which makes for great versatility in how they respond to their customers. They may be coffee shops, bars, local beauty parlours, and other common gathering places. They are a dying breed, especially in areas of rapid new growth where fast food and franchise heaven has taken over. Third places have a slower pace, no seating time limits, and an affordable reason to stop by on a very regular basis with a good chance of seeing some familiar faces.

Kathryn's Restaurant is a 'third place' for many of us. Donna goes for coffee most mornings and is greeted by the staff who know her well. Many co-operative members drop by for the occasional meal, and sit together with whomever they see. John helps out there in his wonderful ways. Caroline Ann drops by whenever she is in the neighbourhood. Some of the families and I find it to be a wonderful place for quiet first interviews with prospective Supporters or roommates. *The Bakery Deli* in Pickering has come to be 'third places' for many people as well. We use it for small meetings, to cater events, and to order those special birthday cakes. Tiffany continues to dream of a time in the future where she might be able to open a tea room to offer a 'third place' in her community to others.

The fifth action is to **preserve professional healing traditions** for those real instances when such a tradition is necessary and would most likely help. In other words, avoid prescribing professional treatment as the panacea of *all* ailments, but instead decide on it carefully and deliberately for when it is truly needed—after other simple and natural remedies have been tried unsuccessfully. When chosen, permit only the minimal intervention needed to alleviate the suffering and stimulate more natural ways to deal with the issues.

People with disabilities are particularly susceptible to receiving drugs and professional treatments as a first resort. This may perhaps rely on an unconscious belief that they are sick or less than whole. However, we have had some wonderful experiences with trying some of the natural alternatives that you or I might well choose for ourselves as a first resort. These include using some massage sessions to ease unbalanced body posture and tension, chiropractic treatment for headache relief, homeopathic remedies for emotional distress, and nutritious meals as part of living well.

The final action is to **cherish place and local economy.** Find local, family-owned or independent stores, restaurants, and businesses and use them and promote them. Discover unique corners in your neighbourhood that define the sense of who you are and frequent them and share them with others in your neighbourhood—make them community spaces.

Partly in our efforts to build community, and partly due to the severe limitations people experience from lack of affordable, accessible transportation options, we use the two local plazas to a great extent. We know that there is something strengthening and fulfilling when we are able to bank, shop, and get our hair cut in places where people greet us by name. When Donna started to look for a nursery school for Matthew, she investigated two local options first and chose one of them. Donna also decided to look for a new doctor she could walk to and linked up with one in a nearby plaza. We have already seen the benefits to her as she can take Matthew on her own for a quick check when she is unsure about something. At the same time, the frequent and positive visits have helped to develop a respectful and helpful relationship between the doctor and this young family.

We have also done our part in helping three people start and manage their own small businesses that also contribute to the local economy in small ways. *The Tiffany Touch* has operated for over five years, at times at a fairly high profile, baking healthy, low-sugar treats suitable for sugar-reduced diets. *J.B. Shredding* is a portable, personal shredding business that provides confidential paper-shredding services in your own home of business. *Rob's Small Parcel Delivery* provides personal courier services in the Pickering Ajax area at competitive rates.

These six actions, as described by David Schwartz strengthen the culture of hospitality in our community. We have, therefore, contributed powerfully to things that make our community strong and welcoming. Our presence is not just a thing to be tolerated, or ignored. Our very presence has injected vitality and welcome into this community. We can feel it. We are a part of it. In many instances, we are the reason for it.

This chapter has been about our growing ability to see our community in its wholeness and its health. In doing so, we also begin to see richness and resources within our community of which we wish to become a great part. Chapter 7 is about what we have learned in the next step of gaining access to those parts of community.

These last three chapters have been about the growing sense of belonging that is shared by the seven people who receive support through the thinking and planning of Deohaeko Support Network. We have come to see that the development of a personally-defined home was the first sense of place for people, the anchoring roots that give them strength to move forward. Relationships that are nurtured and safeguarded by attentive circles add to people's confidence and strength in their place in community. A sense of home and a growing number of relationships allow people to move more freely and strongly to find welcoming places in community, and to deepen the potential of these spaces for all with their presence. These are strong, positive signs of entrenchment. We have all benefited from these experiences. The next group of chapters will show what we are able to further accomplish with our growing pack of tools, strategies and ideas—all derived from experience.

Section 3
Tools, Strategies, Ideas to Work the Soil

During the first phase of our lives within the co-operative and wider communities, we focused on the basics and did well. People were present, they were with typical and valued citizens (most of them, but not all, family members, new neighbours and paid Supporters), and we were helping people do some interesting things with their time. Then we entered into the next phase.

In this next phase we wanted people to belong and to welcome others. We wanted them to be surrounded by real friends and allies of many kinds. We wanted strong life-defining roles that reflect who they were and how they wanted to live in and contribute to our communities. This has been our new challenge.

Over the past seven years, we have had a chance to deepen and learn and protect our gains and move ahead. We have learned that we never stop having to think and plan. The lessons that we learned about support, about connections, about community and about belonging that were described in our first book, *We Come Bearing Gifts,* are still relevant today. We have to keep repeating those beginning steps all over again—every time we hire a new Supporter, every time we want to help someone explore a new community role, every time a major change hits a family and the future changes yet again.

At the same time as having to repeat the basic moves thoughtfully over and over again, we also have to be conscious of finding ways to dig deeper to new levels. This next section is about our conscious efforts to encourage such opportunities and to build on them when they happen.

One of our deepest beliefs is that our sons and daughters are safer and more likely to be living good lives when they are in relationship with others in community who choose to spend their time with them. A second deep belief is that our communities are stronger and better places for us all when we learn how to welcome, accept and honour the gifts of our most vulnerable members. Our sons and daughters' presence teaches our communities to find new depths of welcome, love and understanding.

These two deeply-held beliefs encourage and challenge us to find new ways for people to come together in community. This section of the book offers ideas, strategies, and tools to 'work the soil or tend the garden'. It is about our transition from a showy garden of bright, attractive, eye-catching annuals to deeply-rooted perennials—the less showy, longer lasting mainstays of any healthy garden. It involves techniques, formats and ideas that seem to work for us in terms of yielding good results, that is, people leading good lives within their community.

Being rooted in the community involves people, place and valued roles. Over the next few chapters we will explore these elements that help people to become community members in the full sense of the word. People are present in familiar and typical ways within their community. They lead interwoven lives among valued others in their community. They hold and are deeply identified with familiar and valued roles within their community. This seems like a simple, fulfilling picture and in many ways, it is. On the other hand, it takes vision, struggling with the tough issues, creativity, and constant vigilance. Let's explore what coming to terms with implementing these elements has meant for us.

Focusing on valued social roles that people can and do hold is one powerful strategy that works really well for us to help people live full and active lives. People relate to each other in terms of the roles that they hold in their lives.

When we think in this way, instead of thinking of someone's week as a looming void to be filled with activities so that the person is busy and not bored, we think of the person as someone who holds many positive roles. These roles, in turn, tell us many things about how they might want to and need to use their time well.

Roles give people busy weeks filled with meaning and purpose. On one level, this makes for an ultimately more satisfying life for the person involved.

On another, perhaps higher level, there is much in a person who is fully engaged in interesting and positive roles that attract and interest other people. Many roles become even more fulfilling when some or all of the associated tasks and activities are shared with other people. This is the most common way that humans in society come to know and care about each other—they recognize a shared interest or characteristic within the person they have come to know, one that transcends the limits of any other differences that may separate them. Chapter 6 helps us to focus on the importance of valued social roles in people's lives.

Chapter 7 is about putting together the things we know in ways that help us to take action, to move forward toward our vision of the future. It's about taking what we know about the importance and the power of positive social roles, and what we know about good, welcoming spaces in community, and working with these vital pieces to ensure that life is good, full and rewarding for the community as a whole. We call this process **building a context for relationship**. We have used the strategies outlined in this practical chapter for years with a great degree of success.

This chapter helps to maintain our focus on relationship. Many of the deepest relationships that our family members within Deohaeko have entered into have come about through family connections, circle members, and parents recognizing and personally encouraging new friendships. A second key element in forging new relationships is providing an opportunity for an individual's own personal attractions to shine once they are assisted to be in the same valued setting on a regular basis holding a familiar and valued role.

The final chapter in this section is about the people who are in formal **support roles** to individuals on their journey into the heart of their own lives. These roles are vital and they make a significant impact upon how the person is able to be a full part of his community. Supportive allies engage in the work of building community and therefore we must come to know them well and select them with great care. We must come to know the limits, the strengths, and the potential for misuse of the supportive allies that may come to play such an integral role in families' lives.

The nature of the developmental delays and impairments of our sons and daughters is such that they will require support to take advantage of many of the opportunities we identify. So it is helpful to look at our experiences with support over the past eight years. We have many struggles, concerns and worries about the vital role that paid support plays in determining how our sons and daughters will live their lives. We worry, too, about our own lack of secure solutions to the problems. We will explore these in Chapter 8, as well as new approaches that we have tried and some ways of thinking about the challenges that have been helpful to us.

However, as much time and energy as we put into treading this pathway with those we love whose vulnerability does not allow them to travel it alone, in the end, it is we who also gain. For this is the very gift that these members bring to the ceremony of their belonging. The gift of their presence presents to our beleaguered communities much needed opportunities to grow acceptance, flexibility and caring in our midst.

This is a practical section of the book, yet we must not forget from where it comes. Without a strong philosophical base, we would be unable to make consistent decisions that push our work in mainly positive directions. Without our basic experiences where we helped people to create home, helped to build trusting relationships with family, friends, neighbours and others, and helped to discover good community spaces, we would be unable to think about manoeuvring or improving on these basics. And without our focus on the person, we might never truly understand how our communities can only be better and stronger when this person is welcomed into daily life.

Chapter 6
How People Live Their Lives

This chapter is about how people actually live their lives—where and how they spend their time and how our principles and beliefs affect our thinking about helping people live good lives. Often we tell stories about people's homes and how central they are to a good life, and about the relationships in people's lives and how they flow from family values or growing circles. We also tell stories about the places in community where people are spending their time and feeling welcome. Our listeners nod attentively during the stories but often move on to a similar set of questions. They want to know the 'hows'. How do we come to help people live their lives? How do we help people to think about or imagine who they might be? How do we come up with the places that people might be, or the things that people might do?

For this chapter, I will examine the ideas and strategies that we use most often to focus on how to help people to live their lives in ways that are full, satisfying, and as interwoven with a rich community of others as possible. We have, of course, used similar thinking in the building of the Rougemount co-operative and the development of its intentional community. We use these ways of thinking and acting to design opportunities for relationship at all points of our work, and to finding some basic, welcoming places within our community. Here we will apply it directly to how people spend their time and live their lives.

What Does She Do with Her Time?

A focus on roles helps us answer the question that many people have, "Yes, but what *does* she do with her time?" The question about how one uses their time is based on pre-conceived ideas about people who have a disability as being one-dimensional, needy, dependent and without the typical involvements that put stress on our lives, but also give them colour and meaning.

A person may be seen as a disabled woman who lives in a lovely co-operative housing apartment with a varied range of paid and family support arrangements, who is financially supported by her disability pension, and who has limited ability to express herself in verbal ways. What does she do with her time may be indeed a valid question. What might such a person do to pass the long hours in her lovely home? In fact, what *could* she do? What could she be *expected* to do?

However, when you know that a person is a small business owner of an enterprise producing delectable baked goods, a co-operative housing member in good standing, a nature and gardening enthusiast, an environmental activist, a burgeoning water colour artist with membership in a local art guild, and a daughter with family responsibilities toward a number of family members, this question would scarcely come into your head! The fact that the woman in question also has a significant disability is only another detail about her life that might cause you to wonder *how* she fills these roles and resulting expectations rather than *what* she does with her time.

The descriptions above in both instances could describe Tiffany Dawe. We choose to think about Tiffany in the second way, with the only remark being that it is far too stark and limited a description! The real Tiffany Dawe holds many more roles than the few outlined in the above paragraph.

So when we sit down to talk about Tiffany's day and her weeks and how they flow, we are inevitably involved in the complex juggling of priorities and commitments that are familiar to most young women in our day. The role that Tiffany is taking on at any given time determines her activities and her priorities. When she is an artist, she has a long list of activities that accompany this role. She may be purchasing supplies, preparing for painting, painting, cleaning up from painting, reviewing past works, choosing art to frame or to make into cards, naming framed pieces, deciding whether or not to take a commission, meeting with other artists, attending art exhibits, exhibiting her own painting, auditing an art class, attending an art course, and many, many other things.

When Tiffany is an environmental activist she may be tending to her demonstration Butterfly Garden at the Rouge Valley Pearse House, sharing her lunch with the lively group of other activists who share the space, researching plants or butterfly details on the internet, helping out creating address labels for future mailings, sitting in on a planning session, photocopying in the office, inviting others out to view her garden, and more.

As a family member, Tiffany might be having a cup of tea with her mother, giving her mother who does not drive a lift to grocery shopping or an appointment, buying a birthday present for her brother, sending or returning email to those busy aunts in Nova Scotia, inviting her mother over to a good meal, or just hanging out together with a cousin from out of town.

For all of her other roles, Tiffany has an equally rich list of activities from which to choose which will help her to fulfill the role and in doing so, use her time well, grow as a person, and engage with other people. How we move into this kind of thinking and planning requires us to turn back to our basic principles.

Social Role Valorization

Social Role Valorization (SRV) theory provides us with a framework that has helped us to understand practical ways in which we can help people to live good lives. By allowing the key elements of SRV to guide us, we have come up with practical answers to most of the 'how' questions that we might ask ourselves.

It is hard for the families of Deohaeko to state strongly enough the impact that the principle of social role valorization has had upon our thinking, planning and assisting the person with a disability to a lead meaningful life. Some of the following ideas and strategies have been some of our most effective ways of answering the questions as to how people would live their lives. Practitioners and teachers of SRV today will understand the extent to which our thinking and approach has been guided by the framework of SRV. Others would do well to study the works and teaching of Wolf Wolfensberger and his associates directly in order to fully understand how this framework can have a positive impact on the work that we do.

The essential ideas of SRV suggest that we pay attention to the social roles that people hold in their lives. Wolfensberger writes in *The Future of Children with Significant Impairments: What Parents Fear and Want, and What They and Others May be Able to Do About It.* (2003):

"...vulnerable people need to hold social roles in society that are valued. Many things can be done that (a) increase the number of positive roles that a vulnerable person gains and holds, (b) increase the value of whatever roles the vulnerable person holds, and (c) decrease the likelihood that a person ends up with social roles that are generally devalued. The reason for this is all very straight forward and obvious: people who hold roles that are socially valued are more likely to be actually valued themselves by others, and others are more likely to do good rather than bad things to people whom they perceive in socially valued roles." (p.43)

Human beings are judging creatures. We continually make judgments about the people we meet, and often act upon these judgments. Social roles are the faces of ourselves that others see and make judgment upon. Our current society values certain attributes (youth, beauty, speed, wealth, productivity, strength, health, etc.) and thus, the people who seem to embody these. People who are seen to have the opposite qualities (old, ugly, slow, unproductive, poor, weak, sick, etc.) are devalued in our society. Social roles give people a way to relate to and understand one another. It is a kind of a shorthand whereby without knowing much about the person, we assume a great deal from the social role we see them to hold.

We take on some roles deliberately and consciously, such as when we choose a certain career. Other roles are given to us by birth (daughter, son) or life circumstances (Canadian citizen, genius, arthritis sufferer). Strong positive roles, such as "healthy child, high school graduate, and employee" reflect the values of our society and are highly valued by most people in our society. People who hold such positive, valued roles are seen and treated as worthy and deserving. They are given a high status and other good things are accorded them quite readily. For example, healthy children who learn well get a good education in our schools. They are often extended many other opportunities to learn and grow, and are therefore, more likely to find a good fit in a career. This makes them more likely to succeed in a future job and earn money to live well in society. When they do meet a few difficulties along the way, they are more apt to find the help they need to solve the problems they face. It is not assumed that they are the problem, but that the problem lies somehow in the environment.

Strong, negative social roles are usually thrust upon people, not chosen. These roles lead others to perceive and judge us in negative ways, and if our negative roles are large and life-defining, then we will not be seen in valued ways, not have a high status in our society, and not be readily given the good things in life. For example, children who have difficulties learning often do not receive an adequate education in our schools. They are quickly seen as slow, incapable or lazy not only in the class where they are performing poorly, but this perception is quickly applied to many or all realms affecting the child. They do not get to explore and benefit from a range of varied opportunities to learn and therefore, are not well-prepared for a good job in the work force. They may not find a good job or make adequate money to live well. They often receive such damage to their self-esteem and ability to maneuver in society that they do not learn to relate well to others and are given less opportunity to do so. The problems that arise and cause them difficulties are seen to rest within themselves rather than being a shortcoming of their environment.

People with disabilities are often assigned many of these negative social roles in our society, including those of eternal child, burden, object of pity, non-human, menace, and others. This is to say, they are *perceived* as such, not they intrinsically *are* these things. Often these are the only strong social roles that the person with a disability is perceived to hold. These powerful social roles are often seen as life-defining because they tend to cloud other positive and typical things about the person. The result is that ordinary people in the community are uncomfortable with this face of the person they meet. This is translated into efforts to ignore, shun, or remove the person from their view. The person lives, then, in a state of heightened vulnerability where all kinds of bad situations may happen to them, but others do not know or do not care to change it for them.

Two kinds of human interactions can positively affect the vulnerability of the disabled person. The first is having one or preferably a number of typical citizens to stand by the person and literally share the status of their highly valued social roles with the disabled person and safeguard his options. In many instances, this is the only effective measure protecting the person and making sure that he enjoys some of the good things in life.

The second kind of helpful human interaction is to help people with disabilities to acquire or hold a range of typical and strong positive social roles in order to balance out or outweigh the negative social roles that cause them so much harm.

Strong, positive roles are a doorway to a familiar place where ordinary people can feel comfortable in getting to know more about the person with a disability. At first glance, people react to each other by recognizing the social role that the other holds. They recognize the familiar and valued social role, and judge the person in more positive ways. These positive roles will not replace the negative roles that are thrust upon people with disabilities in our society. But strong, positive roles will lend a balance to others' views about the person. They will ensure that some good messages about the person are conveyed to others, a reminder that this person has more in common than we might at first think. These strong positive roles can hold off the immediate negative judgment and provide opportunities for engagement and relationship. They may still perceive some or all of the negative roles, but these are now mitigated.

For example, a person with a disability can be perceived as a child, a burden or an object of pity. When that same person meets others and is wearing a Toronto Maple Leafs jacket, carrying the keys to their own apartment, and talking about their day at work, others are able to see common, familiar roles (e.g., Leafs fan, tenant, employee) that stand up to the negative roles of the person first seen.

This information and understanding of the power of social roles in our lives has provided us with a way to think about how to help people live lives that are more like those of their peers who automatically enjoy a more valued status in our communities, and therefore live interesting, rich and connected lives.

Recognizing Social Roles

For our discussions, it was helpful to have in mind the range of negative roles identified by Wolf Wolfensberger in his earlier work, as well as the areas of life in which positive roles might be held.

Wolfensberger writes about the common life experiences of people who are devalued in our society. He notes that people are impaired, and that the impairment is a seen as a negative fact about the person. (Remember that as individuals many of us do not agree with the societal view, but we know it is there, nonetheless). The person is seen as belonging to a group or class of people in society who are less valued. They are rejected in many ways by society systematically as well as individually. As a consequence of the devaluation and rejection, the person is "given a role identity that confirms and justifies society's ascription of low value or worth to the person" (p.14).

Some of the major common negative social roles into which members of societal devalued groups are apt to be cast are as follows. The person can be seen as *subhuman or non-human,* seen as less than human in some way, including as more like an animal, or even a vegetable than as a full person. Think of the many times we witness people talking about a person in negative ways in their presence, as if she were not there or as if it did not matter what she may hear.

They can be seen as an *object of dread* or a menace where their very presence causes fear in others, who perceive them as a threat. Think about times when we notice someone cross the street so they do not have to pass by a person with a disability. Think about how many people back away from touching a person with a disability, even as casually as shaking hands.

They can be seen as an *object of ridicule* where they are teased or tormented for other people's amusement. Think of snickers that you see from teenagers at other people's expense, or the endless jokes involving people of low intellect.

They can be seen as an *object of pity* where people always feel sorry for them and do not perceive that they have anything to contribute to society. This leads to being seen as a *burden of charity* where people grudgingly look after the person, but in a minimal way and without seeing the whole person. Think of how often others assume that second best is good enough for your family member, how atypical it is to see people with disabilities fashionably dressed or possessing the latest in household possessions.

They can be seen as a *holy innocent* where they are seen to do no wrong, but also incapable of responsibility or accountability. Think of times when a young person with a disability might take something in a store, and your efforts at restitution as a natural consequence are waved away.

They are often seen as a *diseased organism* even when they are quite healthy in body, and this leads to medical or treatment interventions for ordinary situations where others would receive non-medical support. Think of how often people with disabilities are given psychotropic drugs as a first answer to upset and distress, rather than searching for obvious medical or emotional reasons.

They can be seen as an *eternal child* and never be accorded the rights and privileges of full adults in society. Think of how often adults with disabilities are patted on the head, taken by the hand, given toys as gifts, and never extended the respect of high expectations. (Adapted and based on *A Brief Introduction to Social Role Valorization* by Wolf Wolfensberger 1988, pp.14-16.)

Again, these are important for us to understand, not in order for us to slot our family member into the most appropriate negative roles, but rather to understand that society already does that to them. We need to recognize which negative roles our family member may be seen to hold, or be at risk of holding. It is helpful, for example, to recognize that Jon's developmental impairment, lack of speech and small stature makes him very vulnerable to being seen as an eternal child. Obviously this would be a big barrier for him to overcome in order to focus on a life full of the aspirations of a young man, including paid work, relationships, and his own home. Recognizing Jon's vulnerability in this area gives those around him opportunity to re-balance this perception. Therefore, he takes great care to wear very typical adult clothing and work at adult jobs.

We also outlined a number of areas of life where similar roles might be grouped together. This visual arrangement of the areas of life to think about has been useful to our thinking fully of the roles that people hold or might hold. It is most often helpful to draw these areas up on large paper to help with planning. These life areas include:

Life Area	Typical Valued Roles	Roles Held Now	Roles To Move Into
Home	homeowner, tenant, co-operative member, roommate, landlord, good neighbour.		
Family	son, daughter, aunt, nephew, grand child, cousin, mother		
Friends and other relationships	friend, best friend, girlfriend, partner, spouse		

Life Area	Typical Valued Roles	Roles Held Now	Roles To Move Into
Work	employee, employer, small business owner, apprentice, professional, co-worker, union member.		
Recreation and leisure	athlete, gardener, knitter, photographer, family historian, singer, artist, sport member		
Learning	student, course participant, co-operative placement, auditor, intern		
Community and civic	voter, politician, campaign volunteer, board member, volunteer, expert, committee member.		
Spiritual	church member, altar guild member, choir member, deacon, altar server		

We realized that many of us, in valuing and respecting our family member from birth, had unconsciously encouraged and supported the positive social roles that people naturally held. Family relationships, the valued status of founding member of the co-operative, and other positive roles had been a central part of people's lives. Social role valorization gave us a chance to make our intuitive actions more conscious, to safeguard our achievements, and encouraged more of the thinking and actions that had led to these successes.

We thought that the ideal picture of the full range of valued social roles that individuals we support held in their life would show us various things. Ideally, we would see some balance between the many realms of life (i.e., work, family, leisure, spiritual, relationship, civic, etc.), with at least some roles in each area. We would see that one held many more positive roles than negative ones. And we would see strength and complexity in the positive roles that one held, so that they would appear solid and not easily lost or taken away.

Then, we began to look at the real lives of our family members. Looking at the full range of social roles showed us some interesting differences that did not so much surprise us as give us something with which to work. First of all, there was often little balance between the different role areas in people's lives. There tended to be fewer work, education, community and relationship roles than other roles. Secondly, there were either a larger number of negative roles, or a few negative roles but these were very strong and clouded many good roles and qualities of the person. Thirdly, although people held many and varied social roles, they were not as many or as varied as for typical people, and many of these were not very strong roles (people did not carry out activities in these roles very much at all).

So we set out to plan for a whole new picture for and with the person. We wanted to acknowledge the negative roles that were thrust upon them and threatened their full participation in community life. We wanted to recognize and enhance the positive roles that were already there to make them as strong and durable as possible. And we wanted to eventually dream with the person about future positive roles that they might hold.

We began to talk to other family members, among ourselves, and within circle gatherings about the social roles that people currently held. We talked about how to deepen these roles and make them even stronger. We began to identify areas where individuals were still very vulnerable to being cast into negative social roles. We began to plan for new social roles for people to take on, social roles that were based, like our own, on each person's unique blend of personality, interests, gifts, and vulnerability. Most importantly, we began to understand that this combination of awareness of current positive social roles and current vulnerabilities was crucial to our being able to both move forward and safeguard against future troubles.

Reacting to Negative Social Roles

For our family members with a disability, being cast into strong, negative roles (e.g., sick person, menace, not worthy, burden, object of pity, less than human, etc.) was a given. We knew that many others in society perceived our family members in these negative ways. We wanted to acknowledge what the particular negative roles were for each person (or what they were at risk of being given) and then find ways to diminish these and make sure that no new ones were given. We began to understand that the reality of these negative roles should not be ignored. Part of safeguarding the lives of our family member would always include understanding their vulnerability.

We recognized several ways that we have always used to protect against the vulnerability of the negative roles that can and will be thrust upon the person. Choosing individual tailored supports rather than programs has been one effective way of safeguarding individuals. When Donna needed to attend pre-natal classes, we looked around and opted for a personal doula who helped her gain all of the information she needed in the way that she learned best. We knew that in a classroom setting, possibly under the eye of public health officials looking for potential problems,

Donna would be vulnerable to being perceived as unable to raise her child. Those who knew Donna over time, and who knew of her considerable accomplishments in her life and her unique ways of learning, felt that there was an excellent chance that she would be a good mother. We knew that we could vouch for her baby's safety, but we didn't need to expose Donna or her child to the negative perceptions of others who did not know her well.

Another way to decrease vulnerability is to work hard at non-verbal ways to give the exact opposite message. Jon is a small man, who is often seen as and treated as a child. His family pays a lot of attention to ensure that the clothes he wears are conservative, high quality options that young professional men might casually wear after work. For a time, Jon was also sporting a neatly trimmed beard to make sure that he was not as easily mistaken as a child.

A third way to decrease vulnerability is through building positive relations with those who might come into closest contact with the person in a vulnerable state. In this way, we are able to give the others more and balancing information about the individual. At Rougemount, Elizabeth has cultivated warm and chatty relations with all of Brenda's neighbours on her floor. At times when Brenda has been upset in her home or hallway, most neighbours feel free to ask Elizabeth some questions when she is around, or to approach a Supporter. This leads to opportunities to explain Brenda's upsets which are almost always around the things in life that annoy us all. For our part, we are continually surprised to learn that most neighbours want to know if Brenda is all right, if there is anything they can do, and to try and figure out the reason for the upset. Only seldom has a neighbour complained about noise or expressed fear. Elizabeth's relationship building has given them a context for understanding who Brenda is.

Another way to balance people's perceptions and to decrease the negative roles in which people may be vulnerable, is to ensure that the same people see that person in more positive moments. The co-operative has afforded us many opportunities for this to happen. For every occasion where a member might see Rob have a seizure by the elevator and think of him as a sick man, they would have ten occasions to meet him crossing the lobby to get his mail, attending a members' meeting, or running an errand for the office. The seizure is one bit of information that others may have gathered about Rob, but there are so many others that its importance is greatly diminished.

Enhancing Positive Social Roles

We have also found ways to make ourselves more aware about various positive social roles that individuals already held. We wanted to deepen and strengthen these roles for and with individuals. One way to do this is to simply refer to them more often and more openly. So we began to refer to John as the Toronto Maple Leaf fan, Caroline Ann as the teaching assistant, Brenda as a founding co-operative member, Donna as a mother, Tiffany as an artist, Jon as a small business owner, and Rob as a courier. This is just a small sample of roles, but it shows the range that is possible. By talking about these roles more often, we were helping people to identify themselves in these ways more solidly. At the same time, we were reminding ourselves of the potential of our family member, and our use of these terms opened up to others some of the common or interesting features of the person they were meeting.

Another way to deepen people's positive social roles is to figure out ways for people to engage in activities derived from those roles more often. The next chapter will explore the full power of this strategy, but for this passage we can state that there are simple ways for people to more fully take on a role that they already possess and enjoy. Individuals who are siblings are not always assisted to explore the full range of activities that sisters and brothers typically enjoy. Birthday and Christmas greetings and gifts are often organized by the parent with the individual signing in rather than making their own effort. It is easy and impactful to help a sister begin to send her own birthday cards and a gift to her brother, to make an occasional telephone call, or to invite a sister over for tea for no apparent reason.

Another example of engaging in more activities to strengthen the role, is Rob in his role of co-operative member. He has been helped to engage in a number of activities that underline this role. He attends General Members' Meetings, runs errands for the co-operative office, attends almost all social events, votes at all meetings, and is the general coordinator of the annual camping event. Rob is well known in the co-operative, and valued for his contributions to co-operative living.

A third way to emphasize a person's positive roles is to pay attention to ways to communicate a valued role non-verbally. These role communicators can refer to clothing, accessories, and ways of describing or talking about a person. All of these can be used to convey messages to others about who this person is. When John goes to work at Burger King, he wears his uniform. When it's a Toronto Maple Leaf game night, he wears his blue Leaf socks. When he's off to an Oshawa Generals game, he wears the team jersey. Although John is shy and reluctant to start a conversation with many of his neighbours, he is telling them about this role and his activities very clearly. In this way, one of his neighbours can be the one to start the conversation in very typical ways. "Hey John, how are those Leafs doing?" is a surefire way to get John to join in for a chat.

By the same token, we spend a lot of time helping people decorate and arrange their apartments in very tasteful reflections of their personalities and interests. It is wonderful to watch new neighbours, new Supporters, visitors who come for tea and others wander around the apartment finding things to chat about with this person that they do not really know. We seldom find that there is "nothing to talk about", even with people who do not speak. Visitors can find all kinds of art, music, posters, hobbies, and other items to be the starting point for conversations.

How Do You Think It Through?

I think that when people ask many of the 'how' questions they want to get a picture of the flow of the planning. We start with a number of assumptions, all of which have been described above. We assume that the person is a unique and wonderful human being who is deserving of a good life, equal to that accorded to those of high status in our society. We, therefore, use the imaginary age-gender peer of high value in our community as the standard against which we measure the options before us. We assume that the person wants a rich, full life such as the ones we might desire for ourselves. We assume that holding a number of strong, positive social roles is a basic requirement for living a satisfying life involving some relationship with other people. It provides a measure of safeguard against the negative roles that the person holds. It provides a measure of positive value toward the good things in life that all people desire.

From this solid basis of reasoned assumption, we begin to ask a question. In the beginning, it is often just the family and myself who begin to ask the question. From there, each family is unique. Some families bring the question to a circle gathering, some families keep the discussion more intimate, and some families open the question to a much larger gathering of friends and acquaintances. The questions may sound like the ones below.

- Who is this person? This is answered in terms of likes, dislikes, skills, gifts, competencies, current negative and positive roles (use chart above in this chapter), and future hopes and dreams.

- What is missing from this person's life? This is often answered in terms of the areas in which the person does not have strong positive roles, or in terms of the lack of relationship in the person's life. When it is answered in terms of lack of relationship, there can almost always be a corresponding lack of positive social role in one or more realms.
- What are the typical roles that age-gender peers in this community hold within this realm?
- Which ones of these have enough potential or interest for us to look at more closely? This is based on interests of the person, details that are already in place (current roles, possible offer).
- What are all of the activities in which people engage when they hold these roles?
- What are the places that people who share this interest or hold this role might frequent?
- What makes sense to try with this person at this time?

When we know each other well, our question may sound more like this: "What does she like? Who are the people in Durham who like to do these things as well, where are they and what might they be doing?"

We might answer that she likes to watch hockey games on television. The people in Durham who like hockey include (at the very least) the hockey fans, the players, the coaches, the volunteers, the announcers, the local franchise owners, the sports writers, the Internet fan club members, the fan club organizers and writers, the hockey memorabilia collectors, and the hockey card collectors. Where are they? They are at the arenas, in sports bars, at home, at friends' homes, at the newspaper office, in the radio station, in front of the computer, at hockey stuff conferences, at stores and sports shops, at factories. They are playing, refereeing, coaching, cheering, cleaning up, announcing games, taking tickets, serving beer, writing stories, collecting statistics, cards and stuff, and much more. Within this wealth of ideas, we can always find a positive social role brimming with activities and places to be that matches well with the heart of the person.

We can use this same process to strengthen and deepen current positive social roles, as well as to develop or explore new ones.

Roles Versus Activities

There are a lot of new ideas to try to keep in focus in the beginning. There are the ways in which a day is full and complete, the individual's personal likes and dislikes, avoiding negative roles, enhancing positive ones, and more. Eventually the juggling led us back to the centrality of valued social roles in people's lives. Although ours was a slow dawning of comprehension, some time back some of us began to feel that the lives of some of the people were becoming filled with meaningful activity. We saw that this was not the experience of everyone and we looked closely to see if we could discover the difference.

It appeared that for some people, holding a positive social role automatically led to meeting many of the items on the list of a meaningful day. The holding of a strong, positive social role naturally led to a more meaningful pattern of living. Tiffany was a small business owner with a number of customers and baking orders coming in regularly. It was quite simple to make sure that she had lots of opportunity to make decisions, learn something, give direction and meet people almost every day. And this was only one of several strong social roles that she held. John was a Toronto Leafs fan and had very different opportunities, but this role led him to make decisions about games to watch and teams to cheer, to contribute his opinions and statistics to others, to share his ideas and opinions with others, and to learn something new about his favourite teams. John also held other strong roles at Burger

King and the restaurant next door—more opportunity to lead a full life.

For other people, however, it was becoming difficult for us to come up with weeks that hung together in meaningful ways and fulfilled the many criteria of things that make a day complete. We could often do so, but it had to be a conscious effort and we had to design the context ourselves. Brenda was home a lot, and it was through daily walks and one-off excursions that we tried to make sure that her time was well spent. Thinking in terms of activities that Brenda liked to do led us to trying to fit those activities into filling her week. Brenda's time lay before us like a schedule that had to be filled out, unlike Tiffany's time where her strong roles dictated what she had to fit into her week. Brenda's likes and dislikes, and daily choices had some impact on what was done, but there was little shape to her week. When we looked back on it, we saw that Brenda's time and how she spent it told us a lot of what she did, but very little about who she was. For Brenda, it was time to turn our thinking back to valued roles.

Brenda's Story

About three years ago, Brenda's Circle gathered to help her think about how to become more involved in her community in a meaningful way. We talked about many of her interests and returned often to talk of Brenda's enjoyment outdoors. She liked to walk, to garden, to clean up messy areas, to camp, to water plants, and to notice things in nature. We knew she was doing a lot of *things*, of activities already in this area, but it did not seem to hang together in any *meaningful* way. She was busy but she was not contributing in ways that anyone could recognize. We had to figure out how could what Brenda *does* (activity) develop into who Brenda *is* (identity).

We all began to open our minds to other possibilities. Someone heard of the new Frenchman's Bay Watershed

Rehabilitation Project (FBWRP) at the waterfront and went to an Open House. It sounded promising—lots of events, keen people, out of doors focus—all the right things. The only problem seemed to be more of the same—lots to do but who to be? Brenda could most easily be a *participant* and *volunteer assistant* at events as they came up, but this was problematic in several ways. One, lots of the events were focused on children, and Brenda is nervous around children—mostly because of her uncanny ability to know when they are about to hurt themselves. It also did not protect Brenda from her ongoing vulnerability of being seen as a child by others. We needed a distinctly adult role.

The second problem was that the events to participate in or to assist with were irregular and sporadic—2 or 3 in one week and then nothing for several weeks. This would not provide a regular routine for Brenda—one with which she would become familiar and comfortable, where she could take on greater responsibility over time as she began to be able to predict what would happen and be more adept at the skills. The ever-changing nature of the events would result in Brenda feeling little control over her part in the whole project. This is especially true for Brenda because time and calendars are difficult concepts for her to grasp. Things that are regular, routine and expected give her much more control and satisfaction over her life. One-time events and changing expectations leave the Supporter in control, rather than Brenda.

The final problem was that neither of these possible roles—participant or volunteer assistant—were very solid, prescriptive and valued roles for Brenda. They would not stand out enough to have others say, "oh, that's what you do! Tell me more!" The roles were positive, but not highly valued—not strong enough to spill over onto other parts of her life and other times of the year.

Still, we loved many aspects of this opportunity and felt there was something there that we just needed to give some time and some thought and allow it to shape and grow a bit more. In retrospect this sitting and waiting and reflecting was an important step. It allowed a more solid, valued and enduring role to come forth.

After a time, we came to think what would a role look like within the Frenchman's Bay Project that *was* solid, highly valued, and would provide a sense of rhythm and routine for Brenda? We began to think that such a role would be rooted in a place rather than the roving nature of the whole Project (the Bay is a very large area). What if Brenda has a regular place to go to and regular events and activities that she took part in at that place? We realized that Brenda might be given or designated a small piece of the Bay, a place to which she might return several times a week performing a range of environmental tasks. This was the role of Environmental Steward. The coordinator of the Frenchman's Bay Project really liked the idea and her enthusiasm and further developing of this idea was further evidence that we were all onto something good.

Now we were getting somewhere! We had a recognized, identifiable role: Environmental Steward. We had a solid community link to give it relevance, real content and status: the Frenchman's Bay Watershed Rehabilitation Project. We had a champion for Brenda within the Project: Patricia Lowe, the Project coordinator. We had a myriad of activities within that role that Brenda could take on both at the site and at home: data collecting, water testing, natural invasive weed control, seed collecting, litter control, and many other things. We had variety and exposure to new experiences: Brenda would still be welcome to participate in the range of one-time workshops and events around the Bay. We had a main place to be (the Westshore site) and other community places to be (the Project office, the City Council, other parks around the Bay, and more). We had an opportunity to make a contribution that was meaningful: for Brenda, for the Project, and for the whole community.

And so, we went forth. Patricia Lowe moved the idea and the role into significantly higher status by insisting that we "do this right". We wrote up a formal proposal with her assistance, which she took to her Committee. She got approval and even called Brenda up to invite her to look at two possible parkland sites to choose between. Brenda chose the Westshore Community site, a small parkland where Amberlea Creek empties into the Bay, with several trails down to the marshes and a grassy bank area. Brenda was invited to City Council to present her proposal and get formal approval from the City to be named as steward of this site. Brenda went to Council and some of us helped with the presentation and slides, some were there for moral support in such a formal atmosphere, and Councillor Dave Ryan helped to smooth the way. This formal presentation to Council in itself was an important step in forging a new role for Brenda and was a formal rite of passage that conveyed to Brenda and the rest of us the importance of her new status. She got onto local television and was a celebrity at home and in her community. This was just a start to the various opportunities and occasions afforded Brenda as a result of her role as Environmental Steward.

Over the next three years, she received volunteer recognition at annual events. Her work includes collecting bird and wild life data, planting wild flowers in regeneration areas, inviting crews of volunteers to help pull invasive weeds every year, checking and cleaning a dozen or so bird boxes around her site, and litter control constantly. Patricia pulled together a large binder divided into the twelve months of the year with various jobs and activities for the whole year. In addition, Brenda has helped with Project mailings in the office, she has attended learning workshops and other larger Project events. This past summer she learned water-testing procedures and tested Amberlea Creek water weekly. We have helped her to keep a binder/photo album of her work that she shows to people that she meets. In the Spring of 2002 Brenda received a special Volunteer Recognition Award at an awards dinner for the Project. She was one of only a handful of top volunteers that shared in this honour. Her plaque and a subsequent letter from her provincial Member of Parliament hang proudly in her living room.

Talking about roles rather than activities forces us to think in broader terms. These were some of the realizations to which we came over time. Planning in terms of activity is simply having something to do. Planning in terms of role embodies a) doing that activity with some pattern to it (a regularity that implies commitment and develops competency), b) doing other related activities, c) sharing that activity in some way with other people (directly, or by mail, etc.) and d) being interested in similar activities.

It also gives us a lot more to talk about. When we think about what a person likes to do (activity), we might think she likes to walk and look at flowers and be outside. We are limited to talking about places to do just that. However, when we think in terms of role, we might think, "this person might like to be a gardener". When we think of a person in a role, we almost immediately think of *activities* that the person in that role might be doing, other *people* with whom they might be involved in that role, various *places* that they might be in, and various *role communicators*, or things about them that tell, in non-verbal ways, who this person is and what they might be doing.

A gardener might be weeding her garden, visiting a neighbour's garden, planting seeds, planning her spring garden in the winter with a seed catalogue, attending a garden society meeting, participating in an agricultural fair, purchasing tools, giving away her produce or flowers, and doing many, many other things. All of these activities take place in lots of different settings. The kinds of things that gardeners might choose to surround themselves with are endless (tools, shoes, jackets, hats, seed catalogues, etc.). The kinds of people that a gardener would meet would include other gardeners, neighbours, passers by, garden or hardware store owners and staff.

Each of these is an area rich in possibility. A person who holds a strong valued role is often involved in a multitude of activities that define that role for her. To some extent, we can all pick and choose which activities will be the way that we engage in that role. A circle or a small group of people can very quickly and effectively come up with a long list of activities for any particular role. This is a good way to get people excited about the possibilities of a new role. Try this with the role of gardener, car enthusiast, or hockey fan. Don't stop before you get at least thirty activities for any one of these.

In much the same way, we can explore the many places in which one might pursue their role more fully. Even the role of homemaker does not have to be only held within the space of one's home. A homemaker might be involved in taking some cooking classes, belonging to a baking exchange, collecting recipes, shopping for household items, attending or holding Tupperware parties, or meeting up for coffee once a week with other homemakers.

Most roles have a number of role communicators that can be used to enhance the role or announce to others the nature of their role. People engage in these games all of the time. Young professionals carry certain kinds of leather attaché cases, wear certain raincoats and carry cell phones in ways that young plumbers do not. Activists wear t-shirts, carry clipboards and petitions, and wear foot wear that lawyers going to court do not. Often role communicators are more or less optional, but we can use them very effectively to enhance the positive roles people hold. Mothers carry pictures of their babies, aunts carry pictures of their nephews, sports fans carry the latest statistics, and busy people carry date books. People who receive supports can be, and are, all of the above. Adding in the accessories just lets a few more people in on the information.

Finally we think that looking at roles changes the activity in which we engage into opportunity for relationship. This approach through roles gives people information, it creates time and a safe space to get to know someone. It emphasizes what is similar between people. This will be the focus of the next chapter, but for here it is enough to remind ourselves that it often comes back to relationship. We find that the right paths often lead us back to deeper discovery about relationship.

Safeguarding Roles

Brenda's ongoing story about her role as environmental steward has been instructive for us. We have learned that resting on our laurels usually means falling backwards for Brenda. We have learned never to let go completely and never to assume that all is going well. This is work. And we have found that it is work that never ends for some of the following reasons:

When the Frenchman's Bay Project coordinator changed rather suddenly, we had little time to prepare and so had to work at forging a whole new relationship with the new coordinator who knew about Brenda and her role, but had not seen it in action. She has had to learn how to accept what Brenda can offer the Project, and we have had to learn how to teach her to expect more. Relationship building is a process that takes months and months.

We need to keep a coordinator-to-coordinator link with the project. Supporter changes are too frequent for the Project coordinator to handle or fully understand. In some ways, frequent Supporter changes may reflect poorly on Brenda and suggest that she is difficult to support. The Project staff is made aware of these changes, but know that our coordinator remains more constant in Brenda's life. This being said, in between Supporters, it is sometimes I as coordinator who needs to keep up the support so that Brenda can continue to provide the Project with its data and activities in a consistent fashion. In the muddle that life can bring, there are times when I think this is the single, most important thing I can do for Brenda at the time.

We need to keep our eyes open for new opportunities. The Project does not easily identify which new tests, procedures, etc. that Brenda might be prepared to learn or do. By the third year, we really tried to figure out contributions that Brenda could make that would help out the Project itself. We tried to imagine what would be most helpful from the Project's point of view, keeping Brenda's interests in mind. As a result, Brenda has helped with several mailings, she took on weekly water testing at her site and emergency back up testing at other sites, she has increased the number of volunteers recruited for invasive weed pulling, and she has begun to attend several more workshop sessions to improve her ability to observe wildlife in ways that the data can be used by the Project.

We know what Brenda is doing but it is hard for others to imagine the scope of what she does, and difficult for Brenda to talk about the details. We try out many ways to let others know what she has been doing—wearing a back pack when she goes to her site as a cue to others that she is going out for different reasons, working on a photo album of her site, and putting a notice in the co-operative newsletter about her recent award.

It is hard to find a Supporter with sufficient environmental knowledge and interest to be able to do the work easily while figuring out how best to support Brenda. We have found out that just because a person is a good Supporter in other ways to Brenda, it does not mean that they are also able and willing to figure out how they can help Brenda make a significant contribution to the Project. We've recently decided to try a new approach. We figure that we can teach people about Brenda and how to provide support—that is what we know about. So, we would look for someone who already knows about the environment and has a proven interest in that kind of work. We also suspected that it is not easy to get paid work in that field, and that this might be an interesting alternative to the right person. As a first try, we have found a environmental science graduate who now supports Brenda to do her work. The quality of Brenda's time at the site has improved dramatically.

Strong, personal relationships are still lacking in this picture. Brenda has good relations with many of the Project people, but we have not yet found a person who has grabbed hold to ensure that Brenda and her role do not sink out of sight. That is still our role. The Project has one permanent staff person and one other part-time, temporary staff. Other people are volunteers and are harder to see on a regular basis. Some faces are becoming more familiar. This needs attention to opportunity. It is a challenging job for a Supporter.

In the context of Brenda's life there are many things that could prevent this role for Brenda from developing. In order for Brenda to do her work well, she requires good, thoughtful support. She needs transportation to the site, and she needs to work with someone who sees the big picture and understands the importance of keeping to a familiar routine where Brenda is in control, as well as the importance of variety and trying new things. But Supporters change for many (often good) reasons, and we must start all over again. Sometimes it takes awhile to find the right person. Always we have to start back at the basics and other opportunities must pass us by. Sometimes troubles in Brenda's larger family mean that this role cannot be given the time and attention that it needs. Only rarely do things stop altogether, but often they are slowed down...by life.

We have learned to try not to stop what we are doing when the changes happen, but rather to keep on going. We must acknowledge that this state of flux is a frequent occurrence in Brenda's life (as in many others), and we need to find ways to move ahead despite the obstacles.

What About Work?

In our production-driven society, it is not surprising, perhaps, that people always ask us about work and work options that we have come to explore and develop for the people connected with Deohaeko. I hope that the above information has provided pretty clear guidelines about how we might proceed on questions of work. Because it is a matter of such clear interest to many people, I will describe the kind of process we might follow in order to explore work ideas.

Sometimes, after a discussion of a person's likes and dislikes, good work ideas seem to arise without much effort and only need to be checked against our standards— making sure that they are typical or highly valued options that valued age-gender peers might take for themselves. If so, it is likely that they will also go far in meeting the list of things that make a day complete or are elements of a good life.

More often, however, we start with trying to understand the range of typical or valued options that a person of the same age and gender might choose in our community. What are the valued ways that young people in Durham Region choose to use their day time hours and contribute to their communities? We find that people typically are employees, other professionals, stay-at-home parents, volunteers, students, part-time workers, small business owners, self-employed artists (visual, music, drama), and community organizers of various kinds. This gives us a broad range of roles from which to choose. Clearly, not everyone is working a 9-5 job and making money. Some other highly valued roles make little or no money, but offer one's time and energy to the community in other ways (volunteering, parenting, organizing).

Once we recognized this, we spent some more time trying to better understand the dreams and desires of the people we support. For some people, getting paid was very important. Other people were interested in work that really reflected their interests. Some were open to returning to school for some further training, but only when that school looked like a college and held some prestige. Some people required a high degree of flexibility to arrange their work hours around health concerns or other priorities.

In the end, people have explored many different work roles. These are ever changing of course, but one snapshot in time showed a picture like this. Tiffany is sole proprietor of *The Tiffany Touch*, a healthy alternatives bakery business, an artist, and a volunteer butterfly gardener with the Rouge Valley. Brenda is environmental steward with the *Frenchman's Bay Watershed Rehabilitation Project*. Jon is owner of J.B. Shredding, a mobile shredding business with four different regular contracts. John is an employee of *Burger King*. Caroline Ann is volunteer teaching assistant at a local school and volunteer with the *Ajax Public Library*. Rob is owner of his own courier company, *Rob's Small Parcel Delivery*, and a volunteer with the Second Chance Wildlife Sanctuary. Donna is a full-time mother, a babysitter in the co-operative, and a Bingo volunteer for a local high school football team.

It is easy to see how these work roles alone would lead to many hours of meaningful involvement in numerous related activities in a variety of settings in the community, and often coming into contact with other people. For many people, these work roles only define a portion of their busy weeks. Suddenly, 'how' someone spends their time becomes a matter of setting priorities within limited time frames, choosing between two very good options, and admitting that not everything can be done this time round. That sounds an awful lot more like the somewhat stressful and certainly colourful lives that are lived by busy, typical and valued folks in our community.

Practical Measuring Sticks in Decision-Making

Part of helping people to live good lives in their community is to help them make many good decisions about what to do with their time, resources and energy.

We are aware of how often in our society our family members with a disability are offered second-rate options and choices in their lives. This may include poor education, poor job support, poor wages and benefits when working, and poor health care when ill. Many people with a disability live on pensions below the poverty line and this fact significantly affects the foods they eat, their leisure and recreation options, and their ability to travel around their community. We wanted to make sure that our family members would enjoy very good opportunities and options as often as possible. One way to ensure this happens is having a general agreement to, and understanding of, using high standards at all times.

We hold the ideal of an (imaginary) age-gender peer living a very good life in our community as the standard measure against which we measure a person's choices, decisions, and future options. This means when we are unsure, we measure our decisions and options against those which might be made by such a person in our community. As much as possible and as soon as possible we try to make sure that life's options for the people we care about emulate this range of highly valued ones. This idea has been very influential in figuring out how to help people explore typical options and make important decisions. This can affect all of the areas of one's life. We can use it to figure out what kinds of roles people typically hold at this stage of their life, what kinds of community places they might frequent, what kinds of clothing and grooming they might enjoy (remember in the highly valued, not fringe, group), how they might decorate their homes, and what kinds of material possessions are valued.

When Rob was looking for work that suited him well, we measured his small business idea, which came from a circle discussion, against the way in which others in their early thirties might choose to earn a living. We knew that our idea measured up favourably and Rob as a small business owner would enjoy a positive role in his community. When Brenda began to buy colourful balls and other children's toys at the local dollar store, we were uneasy with the way in which this activity played into to the tendency for others to see her as a child. However, when we helped her to see that she could pass these things along to 2-year old Matthew, she delighted in her new role of adult friend to a small boy. She talked about Matthew at the store as she bought various items, and then she was seen as one of the many adults in the store buying for the children they loved.

We find ourselves shocked at times by our own willingness and the willingness of others to allow much poorer options to be meted out to our family members. It is necessary to remind ourselves from time to time that these things do matter. Other people will make judgments about our family members and those judgments will have real consequences in their lives. We need to choose the most valued options as much as possible. Firstly, because we love and care for this family member dearly and wish for them the good things in life. Second, because these choices may help tip the balance in favour of how this person is seen and treated by others.

Another concept that helps us to measure our options is to choose the most highly valued option available. If our family member is at risk at being perceived and treated in negative ways in the first place (which is almost always the case), we should 'bend over backwards' to ensure that we choose the *most valued* option available, rather than a merely typical option. We have thought about this when we have tried to make sure that Tiffany is more than just a volunteer at the Rouge Valley. She is, in fact, the Butterfly Gardener of the demonstration butterfly garden. This latter is certainly a more clear, positive and enhancing choice. Brenda is environmental steward (by City Council decree, no less) of her site on Frenchman's Bay. When Jon received money to get a new bed, he was helped to purchase a large four-poster metal bed fit for a king, rather than a low-end bed that he might have been expected to settle for. When people visit Jon and pass by his bedroom, they cannot help but be impressed by his bed and the message it conveys about Jon's worth.

A measure that helps us to ensure quality in all of our choices and ensures that we continually aim high is our own definition of 'the good things in life'. We clarified for ourselves early on the things that we felt made for a good life for ourselves. We thought about the things that would make for a wonderful, complete day for ourselves and for anyone else, and then we thought about the things that would make for a good life more generally. These definitions for ourselves are written out in Chapter 2, but it is a worthwhile exercise for anyone to do for themselves as well. Without reiterating these lists again, it is important to note that they also form part of the standard for assisting people to dream of, describe, and begin to build their own good lives.

Our approach this far brings us to a planning context with practical ways of measuring our work and holding up choices and decisions to high standards. This context includes the importance of valued social roles, the standard of highly valued age-gender peers in community, and the knowledge of the kinds of things that make for full, rich lives for all of us. Within this context, the planning and discussion occurs that leads to decisions (made by the persons themselves with support) about how people will lead their lives.

Who's in Control?

At some point in our discussion with others about holding high standards with which to plan and make decisions, we usually hear from someone in the group we are addressing, reacting to what they think they are hearing about individuals having choice in their lives. They hear us talk about choosing the more valued options, and holding a high standard, and they believe that we have taken choice and control away from individuals altogether. This could not be farther from the truth.

We are thrusting unwanted roles upon the person, but rather highlighting positive roles that are already in place (son, brother), strengthening chosen roles that are perhaps overshadowed or not held very strongly (changing occasional church goer to church member or altar guild member), or inviting people to take on positive, valued social roles that reflect a passion or interest that they already have and may want to share with others (long distance runner, artist). People who have had many typical and positive life experiences take on and deepen new roles all the time. Our work is to help vulnerable people do the same with the assistance and support they require for many of life's endeavours.

The people supported within Deohaeko are involved in decisions affecting their lives on a daily basis. They are involved in most of the details governing their support, their roles and daily activities, and their relationship with others.

However, we are aware that limited life experiences have meant to each individual that they may not be aware of the full range of options open to them. If we continually acquiesce to help people choose from among the options they already know, how will they explore the options that many of us with greater experience would readily prefer? Perhaps, in the end, they will not choose that option after all, but their decision will be based on a genuine range of options most of us would prefer rather than the narrow list they already know.

Time and again, we realize that individuals know, choose and prefer high quality when they experience it. Holding up high standards is a way for us to keep on offering high quality options. Sometimes, these will not be the options finally chosen, but most often they are.

Another point that we keep in mind is that many of us make long range decisions (better health, making a major purchase, starting a new career), which require some short term hardship in order to achieve our goal. This is no different for the people we support. Like us, they need encouragement to stick to their goals and dreams, not a flippant "if that's your choice" comment to abandon the long term after some initial difficulties.

Jon may spend his day making decisions about what to have for breakfast, when to leave for his workday, on what to spend his money that week, whom to invite for dinner, and much more. But he is also encouraged to finish up the shredding job he has committed to for the day, asked to select an adult music cassette at the library along with one of children's music, and assisted to arrange his clothing so that he looks sharp and fashionable. The first group of decisions are made within areas where Jon knows a full range of the options open to him and can make his own decision. The Supporter simply follows and supports Jon's decisions. The second group of decisions are areas where Jon lacks experience and perhaps ability to foresee what positive outcomes will result from finishing his work, keeping a commitment, making some adult recreation choices, and presenting himself well. The Supporter with a greater range of experience and understanding the benefit of high standards gently encourages Jon to make these more enhancing decisions for himself.

How Do You Know When It Is Working?

We have chosen not to go into the details of how to support people in new and emerging roles in this book. Supporting a person well is so much more a question of approach, general values and principles and deep thinking than it is of taking specific steps, that it is better for people to struggle with the bigger questions themselves. There is a time and place for people with experience and questions to discuss the finer points of good support, but not in this book.

All the same, there are a few helpful things to say about helping a support person or family or circle judge whether or not things are working well for the individual. The overall purpose of helping people to recognize and deepen, or identify and develop strong valued roles in their community is for the deeper meaning and sense of belonging that this can bring to their lives. People are safer and a little less vulnerable when they hold strong valued roles. People are more apt to be surrounded by typical valued citizens who may stand up for them in times of trouble. People are more likely to develop deep relationships when they are in situations where others in the community can come to know and understand them. People are more likely to find meaning and satisfaction in their lives when they hold valued roles where they can make a contribution to the rest of their community.

There are a series of questions we can ask ourselves to find out if our efforts are working or whether we need to change some of our ideas, strategies or approaches. I find these questions to be most helpful. This is not a formal assessment and there is no indication that if you score less than two 'yes' answers that you must begin again. Rather these questions are a stepping off point for a deeper discussion with others who care.

Is there a satisfying contribution being made? Is the individual able to make an identifiable contribution through the role that he holds? This contribution needs to recognized by the person themselves, and by the party to whom it is made. It needs to be obvious to them. The contribution should be seen as valuable (helpful, timesaving, resource-saving) by the other party. It is helpful if the contribution I one that the individual can tell others about. Finally, the individual should feel good about his contribution.

Is there learning happening? Is there an opportunity to learn new skills, practice skills that one already has, or offer the gifts that one brings? This includes opportunities to learn about work life, about relationships, about getting to and from the place, and about keeping commitments and routines.

Is there a sense of pride present? This is directly related to the two questions above. People feel a sense of pride when they know that they are making a welcome contribution and when they know that they are learning things by being present in that situation. There is also a sense of pride when people feel that they belong in a given place. When a person walks in and they are greeted by name, reminded of their worth, and offered a few moments of personal exchange— especially in a public way—they feel proud to belong.

Is there relationship building happening? There is a whole range of typical and appropriate relationships that may develop when people are in places where they hold strong, valued roles. In the beginning, congenial welcoming relations may develop among a group of workers, volunteers, or organizers. Over time, this may deepen between people who see each other and share an interest or work more frequently. Finally, some of these relationships may extend beyond the original meeting place. For the individual you are thinking about, are any of these happening?

Is it leading to more opportunities? The best situations are the ones that spontaneously lead to more opportunities in many ways. Perhaps there is an increase in the number of tasks or contributions that the person can make. Perhaps there are a few more people that they come into contact with and have a chance to develop deeper relationships. Perhaps the experiences that they have lead the individual to think about other or related interests that they have or want to explore. Perhaps the situation is one that the support person begins to think of many new ways to deepen the role and strengthen the relationship between the people present. If nothing seems to be happening, the situation might need more exploration.

Is there joy? Does the individual approach their time in that role or situation with anticipation and joy? This includes talking about their tasks, ideas, or items related to the role with great enthusiasm. This could also show up as a willingness to show others photos or other evidence of the work they do in that role. Sometimes it is the people that individuals identify with great joy. This may happen in anticipation of the time or as they enter into the spaces or opportunities that the role affords them. Look for joy.

Caroline Ann worked for five years at the Montessori School across the street from Rougemount. At the end of the first few months I went to visit her with these questions in mind. She met me at the front door and entered with a bounce in her step. She stopped in to say hello to the secretary and to Nicola, the principal and the person responsible for Caroline Ann's welcome in the school. She looked into the room where she usually does some envelope stuffing. "Oh, they forgot to give me envelopes" she quickly ascertained with quiet confidence, "I'll have to get some." However, first she told me that she had to plan her day. She obviously had developed a routine which included touring the school when she first arrived, stopping to say hello to the French teacher, Madame, and spending a few moments in two different classrooms. In each one, she stopped to put her hand on a child's head to ask, "What's wrong? Can I help?" Next, she went to look in at the school play and then reminded herself, "Can't stay—I've got to get the office work done."

My impression with Caroline Ann's presence at the school was this was a place where she loved to be. People welcomed her and she had many different people to greet herself. She had jobs to do which she knew she did well, and she felt pride in the jobs that she did, her ability to be welcomed throughout the school, and the freedom she had to make her own routine. Teachers and staff thanked her for various efforts that she made. I saw contribution, pride, learning, satisfaction, future opportunities, and most certainly, joy.

Chapter 7
Building a Context for Relationship

We have come to better understand many of the elements that make the lives of our family members rich and fulfilling. These include a good home, a growing number of family and other relationships, a number of positive, valued roles, and places of welcome in the community. We know that a focus on personal, committed relationships as a filter through which we view all of our work is a strong safeguard for the future.

In our work, we discover that one of the biggest challenges is putting it all together, that is, taking all of our knowledge and experience and using it well to assist people to live good lives within their community. We know that a good life is a life of connection, belonging, and contribution all in relationship with others. We have learned that while all of these characteristics of a good life are highly desirable, they can only be somewhat influenced but not fully controlled by our efforts.

This is especially true for relationship. It is not within the realm of human endeavour to create relationship. *We cannot create relationship, but we can certainly recognize, encourage, and design opportunities in which the miracle of relationship is more likely to occur.* This is the lightening rod statement within our approach to helping people to live good lives. We cannot create relationships which safeguard their lives, but we can help people to be present and contributing members of their community in ways that will encourage relationships to occur. We can assist people to hold and contribute with a number of strong positive roles. We can ensure that people are present in positive ways in valued community settings. We can make sure they meet regularly with others who share their interests.

I have come to call this process building a context for relationship. This chapter provides some ideas and strategies to help sort through the complexities of building a context for relationship in daily life.

In the end, if personal, committed relationships do not happen, people's time will still not be wasted. Holding positive roles, finding welcoming community spaces, and entering into congenial relationships with others present are all things that still bring a good life for people, and more importantly, provide a continual springboard for new opportunities for relationship to grow and deepen.

We all must have a clear understanding about the purpose of our work in this area. First of all, it is fulfilling for people as individuals, and better for our society as a whole, when all of its members are included. Secondly, being involved in relationship within the community is always a better safeguard for the individual than other options. And so, our overall purpose must include both a desire for a better future for both individual and community, and a desire to safeguard the vulnerabilities of the individual. We are trying to afford the opportunity for two people to enter into relationship, for their mutual benefit. The potential for the relationship is that it can make life better for both partners, and for the community itself. It's not very complicated—although it is also not necessarily easy!

A Context for Relationship

Designing a context for a good life, that includes a range of mutual relationships, is based on the following understanding:

1. We may desire, but cannot control, the development of relationship in people's lives. We can greatly influence how, when and where a person spends their time and follows their interests in community. This will deepen

the person's sense of belonging in community and build opportunities and invitation for relationship to grow.

2. We must know about and be able to help the person access community *places*.
3. We must assist the person to be ***present*** in such community places.
4. We must enable and encourage the person to hold a valued *role* in those community spaces.
5. There must be other ***people*** present and available in those community spaces.

This is the context in which relationship is more likely to occur. Our job as family members, planners, and others who care, is to discover, design and build situations where all of these elements of the context are in place as often as possible.

Each one of these elements has important defining **characteristics** which must be understood and in place in order to have the best possible foundation. Each has a **key task** that is assigned to us who help make it happen, and a set of **skills and strategies** that are essential to doing the task well.

Defining Characteristics

Community Places

Community places are spaces accessible to valued, typical members of your community. Note here that sometimes 'place' refers to a physical locality, e.g., a library, the hockey arena, and so on. However, most importantly, 'places' refers to the grouping or gathering of like-minded individuals. For example, the physical place where the local naturalists gather may, in fact, be a schoolroom, but we would say that the local Naturalist Club is the place where people who share a common interest in the natural environment meet.

There are several defining characteristics of community places that will help determine whether it will be a good community space for our purposes. One, it needs to be a place that most upstanding members of the community are **familiar** with, hold in high regard, and would typically use for themselves. We call these typical, valued community places. They would include most local sporting clubs and associations, art guilds, many places of work, and other common community gathering places.

The second defining characteristic of the community spaces that you must come to know is that they must be **typical,** valued community places for people of the same age, same gender, and same cultural tradition of the person with whom you are planning. When you go to have a look at the place (and nothing is as good as seeing for yourself), ask yourself, "Who comes here?" Generally, if you are planning together with a young man in his twenties around an interest in textiles, you will want to gravitate toward community places where other young adult enthusiasts may gather. Therefore, the local church which offers rug hooking to older women on a week day morning would not be a highly valued community space for this young man. However, the local college fine arts program with young people experimenting in textiles might be just the place to check out.

The third defining characteristic of the community spaces you wish to consider is that they must **reflect the person** in some way. There must be a positive link between the person and the place or group which you are viewing. This can be a common interest already expressed by the person, or a group of people who share some positive attributes, such a group of single moms who are at home raising their children. Another workable link is a person who is curious and simply wants to explore this particular community place. The reasons for thinking there would be a good match for this person should be positive and based on your knowledge of the person. You might choose the place because it is quiet, reflective and might be a place where others might talk quietly with the person. You might choose the place because it is a hub of activity and the person with whom you plan is a keen observer who loves to be in the middle of things.

All of these reasons for choosing this particular community place should be shared with other people in the setting. These are positive reasons that others who choose that space will understand, and the similarity with this new person will be underscored.

A fourth characteristic of the community space is that it must be **accessible**. That is, the person must be able to get there fairly easily. For some people, this means that the space must be accessible by transit, by Handi-Trans, or other public means. For others, it means that the Supporter has a vehicle and is available to drive on a regular basis. For others still, it means that the person can walk there, or can be accompanied by members of his circle. The community space must also be as physically accessible as the person requires for their mobility of the site. For some people, no physical accommodation is necessary. For others, it means wheel chair ramps and accessible washrooms. Think about the person who might begin to come to this particular space and what 'accessible' might mean for him or her.

Finally and just as important, the community place should have an air of **welcome** about it. This is different from the first characteristic in that a place can be clean, new, beautiful and frequented by many other valued citizens. However, if it is impersonal and unable to welcome people as individuals, it may not be the most desirable community space for us. Earlier in this book, (Chapter 5), we used David Schwartz's term 'vernacular culture' to describe places that are still able to welcome, acknowledge and relate to people as unique individuals. We need to look for this in community spaces that we are investigating.

We cannot judge by appearances alone because many times an air of welcome can be exuded by a single heart-warming individual even in an otherwise cool environment. However, we need to look for welcoming people and welcoming interior environments. We need to feel that this is a place where we can make a mistake and it will be taken in stride. We need to find places where individuals reign, and conformity takes a back seat.

When we choose community places well, the person acquires yet another place to set down the roots that bind him to community and make him feel a part of the whole. Potentially, the community space becomes a container to hold the possibility of new relationship. Even when the deeper relationships do not happen (or cannot be seen right now), it is a good thing for people who were once on the margins of society to have a growing number of welcoming places to be in community.

Awhile ago, we were helping Jon to explore the possibility of working at Canada's Wonderland. Jon loves thrilling roller coaster and other rides, and the highlight of summer was his trips to Canada's Wonderland, about one and a half-hour's drive away. We spent quite a bit of time finding the right people to talk to and interview at the theme park. We figured out a number of strong ways in which he could take a role and make a contribution at the park. In the end, our efforts went nowhere and this opportunity did not come to be. In retrospect, it is interesting to evaluate our efforts against the characteristics for a community place as outlined above. Yes, Canada's Wonderland is a valued community setting, and it is a place where many people of Jon's age and gender spend their time. It is also a place that reflects one of the passions in his life (thrilling rides). However, it became clear that the distance of the theme park from Jon's home would make it difficult for him to be a very frequent presence in the park. Even once a week would have been a difficulty for us to arrange consistently, and then, the theme park closes down for the whole winter session. It is now clear that this would have been a difficult place for Jon to be at frequently or even predictably. The winter break followed by potentially a whole new slate of staff in the spring would make it a less than welcoming and ideal location over the long run. Finally, while we were cordially welcomed during our two visits to the staff of Canada's Wonderland neither situation was one where Jon could possibly hang out and get to know anyone over time. We never did discover the smaller spaces within the theme park where people talk and get to know one another. The park as a whole and the formal offices we went into were not places that could meet any of our characteristics for a suitable context for relationship. It is clearer now why this situation did not work out for us at all.

At one time, we assisted Donna and Matthew to begin to attend a small church nearby. After some thought, we felt it was a good match for Donna. It was a typical, well-known church held in high esteem in the community. Many other young families seemed to attend the church. In the end, there were two Sunday services from which to choose, and Donna was assisted to attend both of these. She quickly told us that the later service—a less formal affair with live music and much singing—was much more to her interest, being a piano player and a music lover. Clearly, all other things being equal, this would be the better community space for her, and the one where it would be more likely that she would meet others who shared even more of her interests. It is a small thing, but we have learned that *it is in the small details that we build community.*

Presence

There are three defining characteristics of being present in community places that have a huge impact on the effectiveness of that presence. If people are not present frequently, predictably, and legitimately, then nothing will happen to build relationships, except that which would have happened by accident or fate anyway.

Frequency is associated with several aspects. In the first place, different community settings demand varying degrees of presence. Joining a skate team (that practices weekly) sets a different standard for frequency of attendance than does coming to the Mayor's annual Christmas skating event (yearly). We need to help the person choose places and events that occur with enough frequency to make an impression (intensity). The experience must be repeated often enough to make a meaningful difference to all participants. There is the potential for a different level of relationship among members of a skate team than there is for a one-time skating event. Generally, it is the community places where people get together at least weekly that will afford the best opportunity for engagement and relationship.

The person must be there frequently enough so that she becomes familiar with the routines and expectations of the place, and so that others become familiar and accustomed to any unique aspects of her presence. Again, this is more likely when we have chosen a community place or grouping where there are frequent opportunities to get together.

The person must be there frequently enough so that she becomes competent in whatever role she comes to hold in that place. Many people, especially people who have an intellectual disability, learn best through doing. The more chances they have to perform the role, the more accomplished they will become.

The person must be there frequently enough so that there is an unconscious assumption that this community place is as important for her as it is for the others choosing to be there. They must copy the attendance patterns of the most valued others present. This forms one of the first common bonds between all people present. All too often, people are assisted to be in a community place with none of the frequency and thus, intensity, that all others are devoting to the group.

Frequency is often accompanied by positive outcomes. Being a frequent participant often leads to an increase in skill level for an individual, which in turn is often noticed by the others and results in greater self-confidence for the individual. A frequent participant may begin to notice other small jobs that they could take on, details that might be missed with haphazard participation. In the same way, frequent participants might begin to be counted on or asked by the others to take on small tasks or activities that enhance the group as a whole.

As a second characteristic of presence, the person must be present **predictably**—that is roughly at the same time and duration cycle as other participants. If the community place that we want to move into in a meaningful way is the local recreation centre it matters not that the person visits there two times per week if he attends different programs on a haphazard basis. It is unlikely that he will be meeting the same people over and over again if he attends without a pattern at all. He needs to attend the same programs on the same days at roughly the same times in order to meet the same people. His presence must become predictable, in order for him to be missed when he is not present. Being missed when you are not present is one of the main indicators that something good is happening is a community space.

For example, choose an aerobics class and attend the same day and time every week. Choose a church and attend the same service every week. This is the only way that people can slowly get to know each other. The aim is to synchronize not with the place itself, just for its own sake, but with the people who frequent that space and who might gradually enter into relationship.

The third defining characteristic of presence is that of **legitimacy.** The person must have a valid, understandable and valued reason for being present. He cannot afford to be seen as not fitting in, not belonging, not having a reason for his presence. Loiterers, strangers and intruders are the words we use for people who fit the above criteria. Such people are rarely welcomed, usually suspect and often rejected by groups. We need to look for obvious, valid, typical, familiar and valued reasons for a person to be present. Thankfully, this has a much easier solution than many of us think. This leads us into the third element required to building a successful context for relationship, and that is the concept of roles.

When we do a good job of helping people to be present in meaningful ways, they become accessible and knowable to others in the group or setting. These are two important aspects of entering into relationship. And even if close, personal relationship does not grow, the individual may bask in another place of belonging where easy, amiable relationships are enjoyed. The individual will feel comfortable, welcomed, and familiar within one more place in his community. The others encountered in this community space in turn will also benefit and grow from his frequent and reliable presence. Consequently, the other participants will likely extend their new understanding and sense of relationship to others in their own community.

Valued Social Roles

Presence is not a spectator sport. Part of helping people to be present is to figure out a way for the person to be active and involved in each community place. The most direct and effective way to do this is to identify a typical, recognizable role for the person to hold. It must be a **typical** role that a valued person of the individual's own age, gender and culture would hold. The best way to think about this is to imagine (or brainstorm with knowledgeable others—often those age, gender culture peers) who people are when they come to that community place. For example, within a swim class one might be a student, an instructor, an assistant to the instructor, a lifeguard in the pool, a pool maintenance person taking care of the deck during class times, a pool and class coordinator, a spectator, and more.

How do you choose the role? First of all identify the obvious, **familiar** and **highly valued** roles. The roles of spectator are often not very valued. Imagine other young people clamouring to take a turn at getting to watch a swim class. That just does not happen. Yet, so often, individuals with disabilities are offered only the role of spectator. Choose the roles that are more active; those that will cause others to look at the person in a new and positive light. Brenda is an environmental steward. Rob is a small package courier. Tiffany is the gardener of the Rouge Valley Butterfly Demonstration garden. We also need to make sure that we are talking about a familiar and recognizable role. If it is an obscure, unknown or possibly made-up role, then it will not be highly valued. When a person's role is not recognizable, then his other more powerful negative roles might be easier for others to see than the positive one.

Next, talk with the individual about these valued roles that seem **interesting or exciting to him or her**. People need to feel that they are in control over the direction of their lives. They need to be truly involved from the start. Sometimes, people do not have the experience necessary to be able to make such decisions. See if you can find a way for them to experience two or three different roles and see which they prefer. For example, in the swimming pool situation it may be possible for the person to be a student in one class, to assist the lifeguard or another swim instructor for another class and to help out with some aspect of coordination (fix up the bulletin board, photocopy class lists, etc.). Note, that in the effort of affording the person a few role experiences you are also dramatically increasing his presence and contribution in this place.

Then ascertain which role would offer the maximum **competent involvement** for the person and the most interaction with other people in the pool area. This is often but not always related to roles where the person already has some skills or qualities to bring to the role.

When we do a good job of helping a person to hold a role that meets all of the criteria above, the stage is set for two people to recognize and connect with each other based on familiar territory. Each person knows and understands the role. The role speaks to the others about things that they can understand. This is an opportunity for relationship to flourish. Within this opportunity, holding a valued role competently among our peers and having a good place to hold that role means that a person's time is well spent and not wasted. Making contributions and reminding others in our community that they do know how to ensure places of welcome—that's the stuff of community.

We may enter this process at different points. We may begin with an individual's interests and explore community spaces where this interest might be explored, shared or broadened. We then choose the community places based on our criteria of what is typical, and valued for age-culture peers. We then think about the valued roles that the person might hold within that context. Tiffany's circle decided that it would be a good idea to pursue her interest in nature, flowers, and wildlife. With only this interest in mind, we thought of local places where one might share these interests and thought of the Rouge Valley and its many groups and associations. We went to visit and learned of their Spreading Wings Butterfly Project. We really liked the community place (the people, the setting, the opportunities to contribute and to be with people), and so went about designing a role that would make sense for Tiffany. This is how the role of gardener of the demonstration butterfly garden came to be.

On the other hand, we may begin with an individual's interests (likes city affairs, being with people, giving out information) and brainstorm typical valued roles that would allow a person to further that interest (canvasser in local elections, sitting on a town committee, planning a city event, etc.).We think about the possible community settings where this could happen (a municipal campaign office, a provincial riding association, etc.), investigate them according to the criteria. This is the process by which Rob came to be a fan of the Ajax Community Orchestra. We wanted to pursue his obvious interest in classical music. We felt that merely attending classical performances around the city would not be a frequent enough or close enough encounter to be meaningful for Rob. We thought that if he could attend the rehearsals of a local orchestra, he would be present frequently enough and in close enough proximity for full enjoyment. We also thought that the orchestra members would get to know Rob better and appreciate his attention in that smaller setting. So, we set out deliberately to find small community orchestra that practiced on a weekly basis and met the other criteria for a good community space.

With either approach, we remain faithful to the criteria that have been established. Many times, things unfold all at the same time. Often, circle members come through with a role idea or a community place idea that needs to be explored. It saves time and energy if we can at least imagine whether or not this opportunity might play itself out while meeting all of the criteria that make a difference. We need to have a thorough understanding of what is important in order to keep it all straight.

People

Finally, a context for a good life that includes opportunity for relationship needs to include the presence of other people who themselves have several specific, defining characteristics. The other people need to be **present** with the same kind of frequency and predictability as the person receiving support. That is, within the community space that we have chosen we must be sure that at least one or more people are present on a consistent, frequent basis.

The other people present must also be **available.** This often involves holding a compatible role—one that allows for the possibility of a relationship to develop. For example, if the person that you have met in the swim class turns out to be a short term visitor from France returning to her country that day, the opportunity for ongoing relationship is much less than for a typical swim class participant who lives in the area. In some situations, other people see themselves in roles that do not easily lend to entering into relationship. In other instances, we need to be able to figure out that the friendly person you meet leaving the change room just as you are entering is not the person who is available and open to deepening the relationship. We need to understand and accept these limitations, help the person respond, enjoy the brief interactions and keep on looking.

This is often a difficult criterion to assess. In the beginning, we find that many of the people we come across in groups, churches, and other places are very busy people. They come flying into the room for the purpose of a meeting or a course and fly out again at the end of it. This is the nature of our society these days. Young parents, in particular, will be hard pressed to find the time to enter into another relationship. But we have found that often busy people make time for things that become important. Busy people who cannot make the time can still be welcoming, genuine people for the time they have allotted. During that time, they may help build the atmosphere for positive things to happen for many people. We have learned not to be turned off by busy people, but to remain constant and available.

Finally the people—or a person present—must be someone **with heart.** We need to begin to recognize who are the people with heart who might be opened to the possibility within relationship. This is the hardest task of all, and I find that I am often wrong with my first guesses. Those on whom I have pinned the greatest hopes have remained as cheery, open but superficial acquaintances, while those to whom I did not give a second thought have had a place deep inside touched by the individual when my back was turned. My best advice is not to engineer this part of the context. Soul mates will find each other given the right context and support—the magic of friendship will take over from there. Let it be, recognize it and support it actively and well.

To summarize, the pieces of the work to be done well include: we must know the person with whom we are planning. We must know and be able to access community places that are highly valued for age, cultural peers. We must be able to assist the person to be present frequently, predictably and legitimately. We must assist the person to hold valued roles that are recognizable and familiar. And we must encounter people in that place who are available and hold compatible roles.

I have found that when we do well in building all of these pieces of a context for a good life and relationship, then something good always happens. At the very least, people find one or more good places to be in community where they are welcomed, where their gifts and contributions are accepted, and people grow in many ways by their very presence. More than that, people are seen to hold valued roles that will safeguard their own vulnerabilities in small ways, and they lead lives of satisfaction and meaning. Even when deep relationships are slow to grow, everyone becomes stronger and more able to co-exist in a varied community.

Key Tasks

Now that all the pieces have been clearly outlined, what is our role? What is the work that we have to do to pull it all together?

I have come to believe that we are called to work in different ways at each stage of this process. It is vital that we understand how our tasks differ at each point in building a context that will enrich people's lives and provide opportunity for relationships to grow. Mistakes are made by meddling in ways that destroy, rather than build, the context we strive to create.

It is our task to *discover* the valued, typical community spaces.

It is our task to *engineer* frequent, legitimate, predictable presence and familiar, valued roles. According to the dictionary, engineering refers to the application of (social) scientific knowledge to the design, building and use of structures. Presence and role are the structural pieces of the context to which we can thoughtfully apply our knowledge of what works and what can be built in place. We can and must engineer presence and roles so that they conform to the defining characteristics that we have identified.

It is our task to *support* the people who are present and hold the relationship. It is being able to see where and when the good people with right heart are available, so that the miracle of friendship might arrive. We also need to recognize how to support this relationship with sensitivity and skill.

We Need to Discover Community Spaces

We must work on discovering the community spaces that will invite people to contribute and belong. We run into trouble when we try to engineer the typical community place for people to gather. That is not discovery, that is engineering. Others in our community engineer or design and actively build such community spaces far better than we do. They have greater expertise in this area, and they often work with a passion for the enterprise that we cannot emulate. As family members, friends and Supporters we might have one or two such passions but we cannot drum up the organizing energy in other areas, simply because the person you support wants to be there. But I find that we often find ourselves trying to do just that.

In the early days at Rougemount, Rob and his circle tried unsuccessfully to hold Friday night movies at the co-operative for members to relax together in an evening. Members happily sent their kids down to watch the movies, and several other members with disabilities appeared for the evenings. But very few of the typical, adult members that we were hoping to attract found time to come out on a Friday evening.

We learned many things from this experience, but perhaps the most important lesson was about our attempts to build opportunities rather than discovering them. We found out that we were offering an evening event that only made sense in our eyes. Most of the other members of the co-operative were glad it was Friday and that they finally had a chance to relax in their own homes. Adding on a new Friday commitment, however fun it might be, was not of interest to them. However, we know that people do like to relax by watching movies, and so instead of engineering this kind of community space, we decided to discover where and when people typically watched a movie. We saw that some people went out to the movies occasionally with friends for a night away, people watched movies with their families within their own apartments as a family activity, people watched movies at home alone or with friends just to pass the time. Many people watched movies at home while doing something else at the same time (cooking, cleaning, eating, sewing). We realized that with a lot less energy than it takes to organize a weekly Friday event, we could discover several different ways that this was occurring naturally. When we switched from making it happen ourselves, to discovering what community members were already making happen, our options leapt from one way of being involved to several. So, Rob still watches movies, but now usually from the comfort of his own or a friend's home. These occasions are more spontaneous, easier to organize and can much more easily adapt to Rob's (or a friend's) sudden illness or last minute disinterest in movie-watching. Incidentally, we also discovered that Rob is not a passionate movie-watcher and we are far better off to put our organizing energies into roles and activities that are more important to Rob.

This example tells a lot about our tendency to want to manage and control the community places rather than to discover them. I see other examples of this all of the time. Sometimes people attempt this reverse integration, based on the idea that if we offer something great and typical, valued members of society will flock to join us. This is rarely true.

Several times in the recent past, I have seen disability-focused groups try to organize art exhibits and invite other artists to join people with disabilities in showing their work. Due to the nature of their disabilities, the artists tend to focus on their art and only partially assist in the organizing of the event. So the people with the passion for art, are not at the visible forefront of the organizing. Those who coordinate are not the artists, and also know little about advertising, coordinating, or holding a really great art show. Their passion is people and how to support them well. So, on the one hand, organizers who are not artists and lack the passion for art, spend a lot of time organizing for an event. On the other, artists are already fully involved in many ways to exhibit their art, and our efforts may look pale in comparison. We would be much better off to find out where and how artists in the community already exhibit their art. Then we can use all of our time and energy in supporting the artists with disabilities to hop on board. Art is an area of passion for many other members of our community and many artists have found ways to express this passion. Our job is to discover where and who in the community holds this passion.

We Need to Engineer Presence and Roles

Once we have discovered a number of good community spaces that meet the criteria that we know will encourage success, we need to turn our attention to figuring out how to best involve the people we support in this community endeavour. It is our task is to engineer frequent, legitimate, predictable presence and familiar, valued roles.

We run into trouble when we try to discover what a person's role might be by simply having the person arrive and figuring it out as we go along. This sends a confusing message to the others occupying that community space. Who is that person? Why do they want to be here? They will only see the disability and not the passion. Our job is not to discover roles and presence, but to be proactive and engineer them. We need to carefully understand the community space and its potential. We need to imagine the range of valued roles available. We need to craft a careful match between the place, the role and the people present. This cannot be left to chance.

In the same way, people's presence within the community situation needs to be thoughtfully engineered. People must be supported to be present regularly, frequently and in such a way that their presence becomes familiar and comfortable. We do everyone an injustice when we help a person commit to being a part of a group with a frequency that we cannot support or maintain. When we support a person well, others in the group may not realize the extent upon which he relies on us to actually attend meetings or classes. His sporadic presence will indicate a lack of interest rather than a lack of support.

There are many things that we can do to engineer effective presence. We can support well from the beginning and look to share that with other group members over time. We know that we can help Donna get to two church services per month, and we have enlisted the support of the minister to help figure out rides and a bit of guidance for another two times per month.

We can commit to a lesser degree of presence (for example bi-weekly instead of weekly), that may or may not mean a lesser role, in order that the person arrives regularly and predictably and enjoys the reputation of being a committed member.

We can support the person being present and learning their role well at first, and then, when less support is required, ask to share transportation and general support with other family or circle members. This can be beneficial, in that it underlines that the true member of the group is the person themselves and not the various people who bring them or support them.

We can support the person well and shift support over time to another member of the community group, until we are mainly providing a transportation role, which can then be met in several ways (taxi, family or circle member drives, a group member drives).

Obviously, it is easier to work on this kind of presence and support among community spaces that endure rather than short-term courses. This is one of the reasons that it is almost always preferable to find long-running opportunities such as clubs, guilds, teams, or drop ins, over short-term classes, workshops and courses. The latter work best for exploring new ideas, but they usually require support from within ourselves for the duration. There is not enough time to work on relationships.

Once we have discovered good community spaces, and have engineered both role and presence in the most effective ways, we need to turn our attention to the opportunities and relationships of the moment. It is our task to support the people who are present and to 'hold' or take temporary responsibility for all of the details that will build the relationship.

We Need to Support People

This is a different task from either discovering or engineering. We run into trouble when we try to engineer the people in the situation. We cannot control people and force the mystery of friendship and attraction. We can simply recognize these situations in the making and employ all our skills to get out of the way and provide invisible, encouraging support.

An important part of our support is to recognize and consider all of the relationships possible in the given situation. This sounds like a tall order and it is. After all, it is the relationships—the links between the people present—that will determine the most important outcomes for the person in this community space. It is helpful to think of the relationships in a very broad way, and to remember that we are not in control of them but rather available to provide support.

By relationship I mean for us to think about all of the positive ways in which the members of the group might interact with each other over time. At the very least, we want to ensure welcome and congenial relations with one or two people of the group. Our role is to figure out who these people might be—sometimes, but not always, the leader and one or two others—and then to support the relationship. When Brenda started a decoupage course at a nearby church, the leader was stiff and formal at first. It was the woman who did the most delicate work, and who needed most to concentrate on what she was doing, that really noticed Brenda, answered all of her questions and led the group to accept the ways in which Brenda was able to be a part of the group.

Once these one or two people have been recognized, we need to support them in their attempts to welcome and draw the person in. In Brenda's situation, I helped Brenda to pay some attention to the woman's work, gave the woman some information in chatty ways about Brenda's other artistic efforts, assisted Brenda to answer some questions that she had about how and where Brenda lived, helped Brenda sit beside her in most classes, and got out of the way for short periods of time. I also tried to find respectful ways to let the woman know that she was connecting with Brenda in a way that didn't often happen so quickly.

Without at least one or two welcoming and congenial relationships developing fairly quickly, the community space will not become one of the places of belonging that we look for in community. However, when we do our work on discovering places, and engineering presence and roles well, we find that this level of relationship is very easy to find. At the next level, we need to look for opportunities for the relationship to carry on without your presence. We need to find the occasion when we know that we can begin to scale back our direct support because it is either not needed, or others in the group will begin to take it over. Even here, we cannot let go of holding the relationship. That is, we must know who the people are, how they interact, and we must be sensitive to their need for more information, a bit of guidance, or re-entering for some support now and again.

Often, within the safe confines of a structured class, an aerobics studio session, or an event with a set beginning and end, many people begin to feel able and willing to take on this role. Tiffany had been going to the next-door aerobics studio with a Supporter for several months, when the owner of the studio, and the instructor for the class Tiffany attended regularly, approached Tiffany and suggested that she did not need support during the class time. She had watched Tiffany for awhile and had come to understand that there was nothing that the Supporter was doing in class that she, herself, could not do more easily. What is typical about this example is that this did not happen overnight. In the beginning, the owner was one of the people who enjoyed a welcoming relationship with Tiffany. We supported this with words, chit-chat, and generally friendly support, focusing on Tiffany the whole time. The next step in this relationship came only several months later.

Other levels of relationship are reached when someone offers the individual a practical kind of assistance outside of the allotted time. Someone may offer a ride, to send along some information that the person is looking for, or a recipe. This needs to be recognized, and many times the support needed to accept the offer is significant. When someone is offering a ride, we must find ways to make sure that the person is ready to go at the appointed time and that all unforeseen barriers are overcome. At times, it may seem easier to give the ride ourselves. It may be easier but it is not better. This, again, is the holding of the relationship, where our greater awareness of the benefits of this offer outweigh what is easiest at the moment. At this point the new relationship still cannot happen without your presence and support, even when you are not visible. When we let things drop here, the relationship usually drops to an earlier level and stays there.

Another level of relationship is when the other member offers her time with the person in other ways outside of the allotted time. This may happen either at the person's instigation, or the member's. If the person is making this offer with support, we must be sure that the time is right for this invitation. These kinds of things often include going for coffee after the meeting, going to a local exhibit that reflects the shared interests of the two, coming over for tea. Most often, in the beginning, the offer includes the support person. This is fine and important, but it is vital that the Supporter proactively thinks of ways not to be the focus of attention. One of the best strategies for doing this is to absent oneself frequently for short periods of time—allowing some private time for a relationship to grow within a context that may feel safer for the other member.

In the fullness of time, there are some opportunities that blossom into friendship. This is when there is a mutual taking of responsibility for the relationship. Invitations are issued in both directions, and there is a sense of give and take. Even though these are too few and far between, it is important to understand that there is a continuing role for someone to continue to hold that relationship. By this, I mean that someone must have an overall sense of the relationship and an ability to know when a period of time has lapsed and it might be the supported person's turn to initiate contact. Someone needs to keep track of reciprocating invitations, recognizing birthdays, buying Christmas gifts, etc. We have found even when people manage their friendships quite independently, this level of careful tracking is helpful in deepening the relationship.

Every once in awhile, the friend obviously and consciously takes over this role of consciously thinking about, tracking, and supporting the relationship. This is the level of personal, committed relationship that will surely keep people safe and included into the future. However, until this level is attained, and for the good that comes out of all relationships that do not attain this level, we need to consciously and thoughtfully take on the task of being aware of and supporting the relationship.

Much more has been written in other places (including *We Come Bearing Gifts*) about how relationships may develop and be encouraged by good, sensitive support. This short passage is mostly to remind us of the importance of the support role in bringing out the full potential of the opportunities that we have designed.

Skills and Strategies

It has been helpful for us to understand that we are called to use different approaches when we are doing the work of building a context for a good life and relationships. We also find that it is helpful to think about and practice the different kinds of skills that are effective at the various phases of this work.

Discovery

Discovery is about curiosity, diligence and observation. We need to learn to see what is in front of our eyes. We read about the fall fair in the newspaper, while understanding deeply about the myriad of groups and interests that are gathered there. This is not just about the fall fair and the opportunity to go and see it when it comes. It is about people who organize, plan, enter the contests, and are fully involved in the fall fair months before it actually takes place. It is like reading a full account of all of the roles and activities which people enjoy who share a very large set of related interests. Anyone who shares some of the same interests is able to join in. What an opportunity!

We need to be able to read the signs around that tell of dynamic community places—the newspapers, newsletters, bulletin boards, and notices. We need to be clipping newspapers, questioning groups of age-gender-culture peers, sorting through our information, and looking at our community as a feast laden table at a buffet.

What do these things tell us about what kinds of things that other people are involved in? People who have a passion do not just do one thing. An artist creates art, but she also is a member of an art group, helps the group put on exhibits, sells tickets, buys supplies, enters competitions, etc. We need to learn to look for what we are seeking. We need to really understand how our community comes together. Who is who and who does what? Where can we go for more information?

Once we know where things happen that are of interest to us (on behalf and with a person who is supported), we need to learn to know when a community place matches with what we are seeking, and when it falls short. When is it workable, and when is it doomed to feel like failure to all involved?

There is a specific set of skills and strategies that we need to call on at this phase. We need to be **curious**. We need to ask ourselves what is the story behind this announcement in the newspaper? We need to be able to **read the signs**. An announcement for a Community Day in the Rouge Valley means there is a dynamic group of people who are working to pull this off, and hoping to attract other like-minded people. This spells opportunity for many people. We need to **see things** differently. If there is a local drama production advertised, we need to see that there must be a local drama group, people preparing the set and costumes, people taking and selling tickets, people writing and printing programs, and people acting as ushers. Which one of these would make most sense for the person with whom we are planning? We need to **ask peers**, people of the same age who share the interest or passion. We need to ask other artists how they are connected, what roles and activities they engage in, and what else is going on in this area for and by local artists.

Engineering

Engineering is all about planning, reflecting back to a greater philosophical framework, taking careful action, evaluating and tinkering. We need to be able **to imagine a presence and a role** that works for the setting. We thought that the Watershed Project was the perfect place for Brenda, but we had to imagine a role that did not yet exist within that project (although it was a common role in other environmental settings).

We need to learn to **tell a compelling story**, introducing a person in terms that are familiar and inviting. We need to begin and end with the gifts and interests of the person with whom we plan. We need to avoid taking on roles, or talking about people, in ways that portray them as objects of pity or burdens.

We need to get good at **asking a question** to which the answer is 'yes!' When Caroline Ann started her work with the Montessori school across the street from Rougemount, we did not ask if the principal Nicola would take on a kind of mentoring role with Caroline. We did not ask that the French teacher take a particular interest in Caroline Ann and help it lead to her signing for the choir. We did, however, say that Caroline Ann is an organized and neat person who is really good at making sure that things around her are also neat and well-organized. We asked if there were any jobs that she could take on where these skills of hers could be used. We asked if, because this was a new place and experience for Caroline Ann, we could put something in place for about 6 weeks and then come together and evaluate it. Right away, Nicola said that they could use a hand with mailing out flyers and letters, with photocopying and with helping the young children put on their hats and coats for playing outside. The mentoring role, and becoming a special assistant to the French teacher, happened along the way, as Caroline Ann grew in her competency and comfort, and others had a chance to get to know her.

We need to be able to **take action** and actually implement our plans. It is important to think ahead and plan, but then we need to stop and focus on the NOW. It is in the now that things happen. It is in the now that the relationship takes place. We can (and should) plan a context for relationships to occur, but we must then carry out that plan. The carrying out of the plan happens in the now with small and dependable steps. One committed person needs to go and find the place, to identify possible valued roles, and to do so in a caring fashion and that can only be done if it is given her full and caring attention (now).

Relationship can only take place in the now. When everything is put into place and the individual joins the group or becomes a part of the community space and carries out the activities of their new role for the first time, it happens in the moment. When, in pursuing their tasks demanded by the place and the role, they come into contact with other people, the nature of that contact is a moment in time. At that point, it is time to stop planning and guessing and time to concentrate on the moment.

This is also why good Supporters are so essential. We can do all of the planning and arranging that we want, but in the end they are often the ones to carry out many of our plans. If they do not do it with heart and focus, the moment is lost. They miss the moment and opportunities right in front of their eyes when they support someone while dwelling on what happened this morning on their way to the pool, or while planning how many stops they will have to make on the way home in order to get all of the errands done.

We also need to be able to look ahead *and* **think about the safeguards** needed in the given situation. We need to find out what the risks might be. When Rob started his small parcel delivery service, we knew there would be days when he would be unable to deliver for his customers as planned. We needed to make sure that customers understood that he offered a dependable, personal touch, Durham-based service, but on occasions he would be unable to handle their rush orders. When this happened he would be sure to let them know so they could make alternate arrangements. For most deliveries, the customers let us know how much flexibility they have in the particular job. Building this flexibility into his small business has been a way of safeguarding the business and Rob's reputation through unpredictable periods of seizure. It's also led to his customers having a greater understanding of some of the challenges that face Rob in his business and increasing their respect for his work.

We need to provide **good support**, which includes supporting the relationships as well as the role and presence of the person. Part of this support is recognizing when there may be an opportunity to deepen the role for the person, and seizing the opportunity. Tiffany had been a gardener of the Butterfly Garden for several years and we began to look for ways for her to remain connected with the Rouge Valley over the winter. It took a long time, but consistent efforts with Supporters to connect with people and understand the work of the Pearse House Centre finally paid off. An astute Supporter noticed a couple of practical ways in which Tiffany could help out the office staff. They photocopied one day, faxed another, and even worked on a member's list database on computer (a first for Tiffany) another day. The Supporter noticed these small jobs every week when they stepped into the house for a break, and offered with Tiffany to do them. Slowly the other staff and volunteers realized that having Tiffany around was helpful to their work. They began to set aside work for Tiffany and a winter volunteer role was created. We have often found that the initial role with which the person enters the community place is only a stepping stone to more meaningful involvement over time. We need to continually shape and deepen people's role and involvement.

We need to be able to look hard and **evaluate** situations truthfully, and then make adjustments accordingly. We need to understand that all situations are evolving, and if they are not evolving for the better and the deeper, they are probably stagnating and slipping backward.

Finally, part of engineering this phase involves **understanding what both parties need and may gain** from the relationship. This may occur at any level of relationship. An art instructor may need acknowledgment of her skills and abilities, and may greatly benefit from a student who believes that she has much to learn. Seeing this mutuality is one of the strategies that lend enthusiasm and faith to our work. We are truly not just doing this work for ourselves and someone we care for, but in the end it is a good thing for others as well. We are not asking for a one-way relationship, but one in which where each person benefits.

Support

Support is all about observation, believing in the magic of friendship, active listening, gentle support strategies and knowing when to fade away.

Support is using the skills of **observation** to see the potential in people's relationships, as well as in the contributions they have to make. It is about standing back and taking time to be conscious about what we think is happening.

Support requires the **ability to exude welcome** and invitation, without taking over from the individual and becoming the main attraction. It requires us to find ways to invite welcome from others and then turn it over to the supported person. It is about being very involved with but not entering into the relationship.

Support is about **redirection** and offering new ways to relate because the culture does not tell us much about this new kind of relationship. People may ignore the presence of a person with a disability for many reasons. When we don't assume that we know the reason, but instead provide a steady, gentle way for the person to be present over time without great demands, this situation often changes. People are often entering unfamiliar territory when they meet a person with a disability. They may not have met a person with a disability due to the extreme segregation that exist in our communities. Past encounters may have been poorly supported and led to embarrassing or painful experiences. Every situation is a chance to try again with a better context and better support. We owe it to the person we support, the person we are meeting, and our hope for our communities to do just that.

Support is about gently offering **interpretation** to the new colleague, acquaintance, or neighbour. We might explain how the person they are just getting to know expresses their interest and enjoyment. We might explain how a person not showing up as promised is not an indication of lack of interest, but rather of poor planning or difficulty in setting priorities (someone else came by at the last minute). Overall, we can interpret unexpected behaviours and mannerisms in matter-of-fact, familiar ways that lead to understanding and acceptance.

Support is about **avoiding typical pitfalls**. We know of many situations where the Supporter assisting the person in the new relationship, becomes the new friend themselves. What begins with an apparent threesome—person, newly-met person, and Supporter—ends up with a twosome that excludes the person with a disability. Tiffany started a weekly ritual of going to the local restaurant for a drink after her aerobics class in the same plaza. She and her Supporter soon struck up a friendly relationship with the waitress at the restaurant who had time on her hands during the quiet afternoon. After many weeks of this, summer came and Tiffany decided to invite her along to a summer barbecue she was having. The waitress accepted quite happily. Tiffany and our own happiness was dimmed somewhat when we realized that the Supporter took time away from her day off to pick this woman up at home and accompany her to the barbecue. Somehow in the middle of it all, the Supporter had gained a new friend, and Tiffany had not.

The other common pitfall is when the Supporter (or whoever is providing support) unwittingly becomes the barrier to friendship or other relationship. This happens when we support a person to get to a community event, and then pay attention only to our own relationship with the individual. I often hear about people going to tree-lighting ceremonies, summer festivals and other active places and then no attention is given to relating to the many other people in attendance. I also hear from people about supporting the person to get to a class, and sitting beside them the entire time for two or three months, and never interacting with the other people in the class. Relationship most often begins to happen in genuine ways in the absence of support people. We try to teach people to find natural ways to absent themselves from giving direct support. We can excuse ourselves to go to the bathroom, to go and find a Kleenex, to go and get some change, to offer to buy coffee for all three, or to get something we forgot in the car/house/down the hall, etc.

Even when people require a great deal of support, it often suffices to leave them with only a brief note of advice to the person they are with. We must be careful to gauge these moments to people who are ready to take them up, but at the same time we must exude faith in their ability to manage for 30 seconds or more. Often, the other person is not required *to do* anything. They can just be together. We find that that these moments with Brenda have a great impact on other people. At times when we support Brenda, it can appear that she requires quite a bit of skill and attention. When we leave her to carry on while we fetch something, it takes most people very little time to figure out that Brenda requires only ordinary answers to her questions and delights in a quiet moment with the other person. This is true for all of the people that we support.

Like good engineering, good support requires **the ability to tell a compelling story**, but one where the new relationship feels the call to write the ending. We need to talk about people (and with people) to describe their lives, interests and how they spend their time. I was reminded how ordinary and natural this process was when recently I sat down and had a cup of tea with a woman I had just met. Our common interest was in being home schooling families. When all the children had scattered, without any conscious thought we spent a few minutes on chitchat and then each gave a thumbnail sketch of our husbands, our children , how we came to home schooling and our general approach. Once we understood these general things about each other, we had many areas that we wanted to talk about in detail. I wonder how often Brenda or Rob gets to start a relationship by giving a positive outline of how they came to this point in their lives? Yet, when we do so, new friends would uncover many topics to ask about their lives. When the people we support cannot give the full story themselves, we need to find respectful, interesting ways to do this for them.

Support is about faith in other people, listening for the words and actions of friendship, and reacting with gentle but solid interactions of support.

There are, then, different skills sets for different stages in building a context for relationship to grow. It makes a difference when we recognize what point we are at and which skills might bring us the best results. It's not always easy, but with conscious effort many of these approaches become second nature to us. Our work is challenging, complex and satisfying. We need to continually be asking ourselves what contributions of skills and gifts we bring to this work.

I want to end this chapter with an example of one way that we can be thoughtful and reflective while pulling all of this complex material together as best we can. I think that we can realize that as we go about our work, there are many parts that I have outlined above, which we do automatically. If we can raise our awareness of our thinking and actions in these areas, and then learn some of the newer ideas and approaches, the result is an achievable, impactful plan of preparation, action and support. That was how it worked in one of Caroline Ann's stories.

A Retreat in Search of Possibilities at the Loretto Centre

Caroline Ann has long had a fascination with Niagara Falls. This is the home of her family on both her mother's and her father's sides. Many fond childhood memories for Caroline Ann lay within the stories of travelling to grandparents, aunts, uncles and cousins for holiday gatherings. The Loretto Centre (formerly a Catholic high school, it is now a Catholic learning and retreat centre) in Niagara Falls is a place for many of its own memories, being the place where Caroline's mother and her two sisters went to high school. It is a place she has been back to visit many times.

Now as an adult, many things have changed for Caroline Ann. Her grandparents are no longer living, many family members live farther apart, and Niagara Falls itself is on an urbanization and building boom spurred on by the new casino. But history and family have deep roots for Caroline Ann and she determinedly finds new ways to regain her hold of joyful memories. She finds that visiting and talking at the graveside to her grandparents in the local cemetery is a worthwhile touchstone during her visits to Niagara Falls. Although painful at times, they also fill her with a sense of peace and right-ness that she carries with her. She rejoices in the fact that her beloved namesake, Aunt Caroline, has returned to Niagara Falls and the Loretto Life Centre. And Caroline Ann has also discovered that she can and does navigate the busy downtown area to discover dollar stores and gift shops that become regular places to visit.

Recently, Helen, Caroline Ann's mother, has wondered about Caroline Ann spending some time at the Loretto Life Centre on a retreat. As family comes and goes, there is a sense that perhaps this centre of spirituality might provide for Caroline Ann a reliable and welcoming place to tie her to this city. I was elected to go along with Caroline Ann for a two-night stay to discover how this might be a community space of welcome and belonging for Caroline Ann.

We know that this centre is a place of rich and honourable history for this city. It holds a valued status to many citizens both inside and outside of Niagara Falls. Within the Catholic Church of which Caroline Ann is a member, the Loretto Centre holds an important role. We can, thus, surmise that the Loretto Centre is a highly valued and typical community space. In addition, Caroline's fondness for the Centre makes it a very inviting place to be in her own eyes.

We know that much of the life and history of the centre revolves around the actions of strong women in the Church who take action to make the world a better place. It is a common and valued practice for middle-aged women to go on retreat for a few days throughout the year. Therefore, the role of retreatant is one that Caroline Ann can enter into easily. She is also the niece of one of the directors of the Centre and this role, together with her family's history with the Centre, gives her many obvious and solid reasons to be at the Centre. Within these roles, Caroline Ann can easily be present on the frequent and predictable basis that good opportunities require.

Within a short time at the Centre, I discover many other details that deepen and accentuate Caroline Ann's connection to the Centre. Firstly, she knows the layout of the Centre and its nooks and crannies intimately. Hers is not an idle curiosity, but a strong love for the history and stories that she knows lies within these walls. She absolutely glows when she discovers a classroom that her mother once frequented. In fact, she ends up bringing some written work down there later on in our stay in order to bask in the memories a bit more deeply. The sisters and the staff of the centre recognize this glow and delight in someone who loves this place as much as they do.

The predictable rhythms and routines of the Centre match Caroline Ann's love of schedule perfectly. She knows exactly when meals will be served and can plan her days easily around these times. She knows that she will find people watching television on the second floor in the evening. There is enough structure here to hold her well. She knows when she can get together with others, and she loves the free space in between these times that allow her some time on her own.

The final element in thinking about the Centre experience is the people she will encounter. At the heart of the Centre is Aunt Caroline who met us at the door, who walked us around the introductions to the other sisters present, and who Caroline Ann could count on seeing casually over the next couple of days. In addition, Aunt Caroline invited us out for dinner one night, and gave us something unexpected to look forward to.

The sisters of the Centre greeted Caroline Ann literally with open arms. They engaged with her immediately in many different ways. Sister Marian and Sister JoAnn immediately made sure that she would join them to watch that night's hockey game (Caroline Ann's favourite spectator sport). Sister Mariana looked up the hockey schedule in detail, and also provided details on visiting the big Skylon Tower tourist attraction. Sister Ursula spent some personal time with Caroline Ann on spiritual matters, as all retreatants do. We were invited to take our meals together with the whole group of sisters who call the Loretto Centre home.

The housekeeping staff also greeted Caroline Ann with hugs and they were delighted to pose with her for a photograph. At her request they also accompanied Caroline Ann to the Centre gym to reminisce about old school teams and shoot a couple of baskets.

Clearly, there are people present and available to Caroline Ann in many wonderful ways.

Within this positive environment, it was wonderful to watch Caroline Ann explore her own possibilities. I had brought my own work with me and deliberately spent little time supporting her to fill her time. After supper on the first evening, she took me on a tour of the Centre and then left me at my room while she went off on her own. It turns out she went off to watch hockey, eat popcorn, and then get assistance to call home from an office telephone.

The next morning, Caroline Ann was prompt for breakfast and joined me for a walk afterwards. We discovered a trail down to the Falls area and Caroline Ann thought that she could do that on her own later on. First of all she had a busy morning that she planned on her own. She went and found a classroom to do some of her own work, on her mother's turf as it were. She then met for a bit with Sister Ursula. Later she came upstairs and listened to her music for an hour as she does everyday no matter where she is. After a good lunch, she went off to the Falls area—emergency telephone number as back up in pocket. She returned over two hours later, red-faced and jubilant from her adventures. She walked and shopped and took photographs. She ran out of film and had to buy a new disposable camera. She had a great time and was impressed with herself for getting out so far (and back so steeply—up the escarpment) on her own.

At 4:00 we joined Aunt Caroline for a drive and dinner. We stopped off at Grandpa Dawson's previous home for pictures and then made our way to the cemetery. Caroline Ann brought flowers for Grandpa Dawson and had a short conversation with him. She placed flowers and a few tears at the graveside of Grandma Dionne and spoke with her at length and with great emotion. We finished off the evening by driving in the October sunshine to Niagara-on-the-Lake for dinner, and returning by full moon light. Before bed, Caroline Ann made the rounds of the Centre hallways, the television room, and a visit to the office to call home.

Is this a place for Caroline Ann to spend some time in the future? Almost certainly. She can be easily present here in a place where the routines, structures, and welcoming people can give her great independence. She has a number of valued, obvious roles to hold. These define her time and give meaning to her activities. There are a number of open, kind and welcoming people who just might be available to greater relationship. As well, there is potential on the road ahead. There are many unexplored roles for Caroline Ann to think about (assistant in the school programming, kitchen aide, dining room help, tour guide, and more). There are a number of people who will encounter Caroline Ann in her glory—when she glows with delight at the rightness of the world. Someone may feel compelled to get to know her just a little bit better.

Will there be a deep and abiding relationship within these walls? That we cannot say. The language of relationship is a mystery. However, as one of many community spaces for Caroline Ann to be a part of during her year, this one has potential.

This is an important story because it illustrates for us the coming together of thoughtful people who wanted to go about planning and thinking with Caroline Ann in good and helpful ways. It shows us what a difference it makes when we apply some structured thinking to the plans that we are able to make with our family members. When we know that some of the basics are in place—community space, presence, a valued role, and good, available people— we can then spend our time thinking about how to maximize each one of these.

Despite all that we know and all we have learned, supporting people well in new relationships is a complex process where success in not guaranteed. Many of us have being doing this for ourselves all of our lives without much conscious thought on the matter. For those who require support, each step can take much thought, care and understanding. However, at the same time, even in moments where circumstances seem very imperfect indeed, opportunity may bloom. Our awareness of the complexity of this process may help us to seize the moments that come before us.

Chapter 8
Supportive Allies

I refer to the people who take on paid roles to support the work of families and the life of individuals as 'supportive allies'. I include coordinators or facilitators, support workers, students and others in this group. The work of building community cannot just be left to very busy families. It must begin to include a range of others who share the dreams. Typical community members who become friends, colleagues and circle members are the first allies who will build a different community with families. But others are needed as well. Supportive allies are those who may bring special talents and gifts, often because their paid role allows them to spend more time to focus on bringing the dreams to reality.

The first half of this chapter is about our experiences with Supporters over the past decade, and the second half focuses on the role of the coordinator.

Supporters

There is much to say about the vanguard of our supportive allies: the direct support workers who are paid for their time. We call them Supporters. Good Supporters are key to our vision of a good life for people who have a disability. When things are going well, their key position should not be too obvious. People are quietly supported to shine in their own homes, be present in valued community settings, and engage meaningfully with others that they connect with in their community. At times of crisis for the individual or family, their presence and gifts are seen more clearly. Families wonder how their sons and daughters, or they, themselves, would ever manage without their skills, insight, and reliable support. When paid support is not going well, we feel the full impact of its lack and understand its key role in the vision acutely.

The following section is about our experiences with Supporters over the past decade. I have described some of the main issues that arise and some ideas that we have found useful to think about in order to deal with them. Part of the discussion is my own analysis or thinking from my position of accompanying families but being once removed from standing in their shoes. Here is some of what I have come to know and think about Supporters over this time.

Finding Supporters

Finding good Supporters has always been a challenge, and we seem to go through cycles when finding any kind of Supporter at all is almost impossible. The families of Deohaeko typically have between sixteen and twenty mostly part-time Supporters working with their seven sons and daughters over the course of the week. Each Supporter only works with one family, usually for a fairly consistent number of hours per week. This can range from 3 to 40 hours per week, depending on the individual situation. However, there are only a few Supporters who spend more than 20 hours per week with a person. Two individuals spend time with only one Supporter each, one individual sees up to six different people every week, and the others lie somewhere between. Many families have enjoyed periods of relative stability with a group of Supporters, and a few families have had periods of constant changeover. It seems that where a group works well together, the whole group endures longer. The challenge for a family undergoing constant change is to find a core Supporter who is determined to stay. This seems to lend stability to the group as subsequent new Supporters begin to settle in for the longer term as well.

Currently there are four Supporters who have been around for almost ten years, and another eight Supporters who have been with families for over three and up to seven years. This is a wonderful track record!

We have examined the profiles of the Supporters who have been around for more than five years (11 individuals), and found that for the most part, these long-term Supporters are women (one is a man). They are between the ages of 30 (25 at the time they started) and 50 and are typically married with families of their own. They tend to have teen aged or grown children. They live with their spouses who often work at full-time jobs with benefits. The additional income from this support work is vital to their family well being for half of them; for the others it is welcomed and necessary but not indispensable for the family. All of these long-term Supporters have experience in making a home, raising children, and working at several kinds of jobs. None of them has a professional degree and one has a certificate specifically to work with people with disabilities. All of these Supporters seem to have a deep interest or passion that they follow in their lives. Two are artists, and others have a demonstrated commitment to minor league football, computers, outdoor life, their own ethnic culture, drama, choir, or church.

On a few occasions we have met with these Supporters as a group to hear their side of the story. They told us that they enjoyed their work most of all because of the bond that they had formed with the person themselves. Next to that they noted that what kept them connected were the satisfaction of doing work that made a difference, the flexibility of the hours, bonds to the parents, and coming to believe in the importance of people with disabilities being part of their community.

This successful profile is one we seek whenever we search for new support. This being said, we look for and find good Supporters in all kinds of places. We ask other Supporters, ask other families, and ask circle members. We post notices at job placement agencies, on college bulletin boards, at schools and on some community boards. We talk to people we know at schools, associations and clubs. We use college placement students and try to hang on to the good ones. At all times, we are aware of the importance of using positive imagery and descriptions to describe the individuals and the work (see Chapter 2).

We continually go through cycles of finding it hard to locate good Supporters. There are times when despite our best efforts and our tried-and-true methods, individuals experience gaps of time between Supporters. Other Supporters for that family, family members, neighbours and others fill in during these times. However, we have found that it is much better to muddle along in this way waiting for the right match, than make a hasty decision with someone unsuitable.

Orientation of New Supporters

We believe that the process of helping new Supporters to understand our approach and our thinking begins at the very first contact. This is the reason we have put much thought into every part of our recruitment and hiring process. Our job postings are carefully worded in order to present a positive and active image of the person requiring support (as outlined in *Telling Our Stories* in Chapter 2), but also in order to call forth positive and desirable qualities of the potential Supporter. The following is an example of this in part of a job posting:

…we would prefer an individual who:
- *Has some experience in providing support to people with disabilities in the community.*
- *Is familiar with the Pickering and Durham Region community.*
- *Is comfortable and articulate in public situations, and can quietly and gently encourage people to get to know each other in new situations.*

- *Is flexible in their approach to getting a job done, and can respond with warmth and humour to many situations.*
- *Is comfortable and interested in introducing this woman to various people they know in the environmental movement in our community.*
- *Has a firm belief that people with disabilities are an integral part of our community, and that communities are stronger when all members are included in meaningful ways.*

Once the person is hired, most families try to ensure that they understand that the initial three months is really an opportunity for all three parties—the new Supporter, the individual receiving support, and the family—to figure out if they would like to work together. In this period, the Supporter needs to learn and understand many things. At the very least, the Supporter will need to learn about:

- Who is this person and how can I best get to know to her directly?
- Where is this person in her life? What are her goals, dreams and aspirations?
- What part of this picture am I to support directly?
- Where has this person been in her life (in broad strokes) and what does this mean for how she feels about her life right now?
- What are the essential strengths and gifts of this person, and how do they relate to how I spend my time with her (i.e., is she to be engaged in one of these roles while I am with her)?
- What are the greatest vulnerabilities of this person and how do they relate to how I spend my time with her?
- What are the daily routines for which we are responsible together? How does this fit into the bigger picture of her day and week?
- Who are the important people in her life and what is my role in maintaining or deepening these relationships?

- With whom do I communicate about our time together (including achievements, insights, concern, questions and problems) and how do I do so?

While these concrete elements of orientation are going on, families must begin another level of discussion and direction. This is aimed at the person coming to understand about some of the basic values and principles that underlie our approach, and how these impact on our day-to-day lives, including their support work. This discussion includes:

- The inherent worth and value of each person as a unique human being.
- It is always preferable to look for options and choices that lead one to community rather than segregation. This is safer and better for the individual; it is better for our community.
- In all that we do, we place a very high value on roles, activities and choices that enhance the likelihood of inviting or strengthening relationship for and with our son or daughter
- When in doubt, choose options that are familiar and valued for well-known, well-liked others of similar age, gender and culture in our community.
- Time is valuable; don't waste it.
- You are here to be with this person in supportive ways. They are always your priority. Casual use of cell phones, making social or other appointments during work time, meeting with other Supporters, wearing distracting clothing (messy, uniform-like, too formal, too casual), or running your own errands are in contradiction to this idea.

These are the very basics of orientation. If the Supporter is unable to grasp these basic facts and understandings of the work, their time with us will be very limited. Understanding and using these basics well will make for a good, competent Supporter that may assist the person to move in good directions.

Dimensions of Support Relationships

Over time, we try to bring the new Supporter to a deeper level of seeing their time and their presence with the person they are supporting. There are different words to describe this way of living, working, and being. Some refer to it as service. In my recent reading I have come across a delightful book by Rachel Naomi Remen, called *My Grandfather's Blessings*, and among many of the gems therein, I found these profound thoughts on service:

> Basically service is about taking life personally, letting the lives that touch yours touch you.... (p. 197)

Another quote draws our attention to the depth of emotions we may touch in our support of another person.

> Many times when we help we do not really serve. Those who help see life differently from those who serve...It is not hard to see the person you are helping as someone weaker than yourself, someone more needy. When we help we become aware of our strength because we are using it. Others become aware of our strength as well and may feel diminished by it. But we do not serve with our strength; we serve with ourselves. We draw from all of our experience....The wholeness in me serves the wholeness in others and the wholeness in life. The wholeness in you is as worthy as the wholeness in me. Service is a relationship between equals....

> Many times my limitations have become the source of my compassion, my wounds have made me gentle with the wounds of other people...

> A helping relationship may incur a sense of debt, but service, like healing, is mutual. Service is free from debt. The wholeness in me is as strengthened as the whole in you. Everyone involved is fortunate to have had the chance to participate. In helping, we may find a sense of

satisfaction; in service we have an experience of gratitude.

The best definition of service I have come across is a single word, BELONGING. Service is the final healing of isolation and loneliness. It is the lived experience of belonging. (pp. 198-200)

Others may call these sentiments 'love', or simply refer to a deep emotion involving elements of joy, caring and respect. I think that when we invite the Supporter to get to know the person in full and true ways, and when we spend lots of time with the Supporter in discussion to ground their increasing knowledge, we are setting the stage and inviting this deep emotion to grow. Whether or not this emotion grows to love that involves freely-given commitment is not able to be known at this point. Love is one of those things that you cannot mandate and you cannot control. But we know that the gifts of our family members with a disability shine best in small, intimate moments over time. When we do our orientation well we are able to offer many moments like this where the mystery of love or deep caring has a chance to grow.

In our own unending love for our family member, we may leap to assumptions about the commitments tied to this deep emotion that precedes love. We may believe the Supporter means to be in the person's life forever. The depths of love are endless, but not everyone will go to the depths. Some Supporters will use the shallow waters of love—a depth of emotion sparked with joy—to deepen their work, to bless the journey they are currently on with this one person. When this happens, it is, in and of itself, good. It is good and right for both the Supporter and the supported person when the hours spent in each other's company are mutually satisfying. The quality of care cannot help but be increased when this happens. Enthusiasm for attaining dreams and goals grows and new creativity is found. The Supporter finds meaningful things to do with their time. The family who comes to know and recognize this spark of caring in the work being done knows that their family member is safe and well-engaged during their times together. There is no promise for the future in this caring interaction, but a deep respect for the present, which is a wonderful quality to find.

Support and Friendship

In the best of all possible worlds, the following is the understandable flow of things. A family seeks and finds a good Supporter. She is reliable, respectful, creative and motivated. They provide solid orientation over a period of months and the Supporter gains the skills and knowledge necessary to helping the person move forward in good ways. Over time, deep respect and caring may grow in that fertile ground. This deep emotion centres the work and the Supporter finds that it matters greatly what is done with the person during their time together and how it is achieved together. The person comes to understand that this Supporter will, indeed, help her achieve one or two of her life dreams. Over more time still, a friendship is forged between the two of them, a friendship that carries a commitment to time and attention beyond the boundaries of paid hours. This commitment is played out when the Supporter moves on to new work, and keeps in touch in concrete, practical and regular ways.

For most of us, however, the saga turns a bit sour around the bottom half. The good Supporter arrives, receives a decent orientation, and makes some reasonable and welcome progress in helping the person with their life. Over a fairly short period of time, perhaps less than three months, the Supporter describes herself as the person's friend and may profess her undying love and commitment to the individual. Perhaps she talks on the telephone with the person, invites them to her wedding, or offers to vacation with them for only a stipend rather than an hourly rate. The two together greatly enjoy their time spent in each other's company—what they do with their time is relatively unimportant because they are having so much fun just hanging out together. Then, suddenly, the Supporter suffers a personal crisis or life-altering event. Perhaps her husband loses his job, or she has a disagreement with the parent of the disabled person, or she decides to go back to school, or she is having a baby, or she is getting married, or she is offered a job with benefits that she cannot refuse. She finds it necessary to leave her support role with this person. She leaves, often with a farewell party and much fanfare and good wishes. She promises to keep in touch with her 'good friend'. After a couple of weeks, she phones once, and a month later she visits once. Then her new life takes over, many other things fill the time that once she spent with the supported person (the baby, the hours of the new job, homework, a new boyfriend, etc.), and she is not heard from again. When the supported person calls to invite her to a special occasion she makes it once or twice and then is gone. What happened? Where is friendship? Where is love? What happened and why is this so distressingly familiar?

This scenario is so familiar to me over the years that I tried to analyze it again and again. It is important to try and figure it out because the experience is so obviously painful to the person who is abandoned. To the best of my understanding this is what I think is happening. I think our seeking and finding the right people needs some further work and attention, but basically I think that we know how to find and welcome Supporters who have the right basic attributes and who are ready and able to learn the basic Supporter requirements over time. I also believe that our group of families knows a lot about the basic orientation and is quite good at helping new Supporters to acquire the new skills and understanding to provide good support to their son or daughter.

What goes wrong happens at about this point. The Supporter who is anxious to be accepted and to do a good job works really hard at the relationship with the individual.

As she comes to see and appreciate the person beyond the façade that is the first encounter, she is entranced by this person. Perhaps she begins to feel a degree of deep emotion unlike any she has felt before. However in our society, we have no words for this outside of the context of friendship, courtship or family relationship. The Supporter has no other language for this but to speak of friendship.

I believe friendship is another entity altogether. Friendship implies love, commitment over the long term, standing by when things get rough, and a quality of durability and longevity. Friendship is unpaid.

What the Supporter feels is that in-the-moment feeling of rightness and goodness that comes from the heart. It may transcend time and involve commitment, but it does not need to. I don't believe the Supporter can possibly mean personal commitment at this stage of the relationship. I think that she, in fact, means "Hey, this person is real and whole and there is something about her that I love to be around. I like to be in her presence. I want things to be good for her while I am here. She makes me feel good about my work, myself, and I want to share that with her."

I think that families need to stop a Supporter in these early stages of talk of friendship and have a deep discussion about what might be going on. I think that we need to tell her that the happiness she feels inside when she is around Tiffany has to do with that special spark that can grow between two people. This may eventually lead to love when true commitment and depth is shown. In the meantime, this spark makes our work even more worthwhile and can lead us to heights of excellence because it will spur us on to take more risks and work harder.

We need to say that while friendship (involving love and commitment) would be certainly welcome in the long run, it is a different thing altogether. Friendship involves commitment, personal sacrifice, and a re-ordering of priorities. The simple fact of the pay cheque muddies the waters so that it is impossible to tell, except in retrospect, if there is a friendship there at all. In these circumstances, we can only look back a year or so after the end of the paid relationship, when the connection is still constant and growing, and say, yes there is a friendship there after all. For the Supporters that remain skeptical, we should keep a running count of the difference between the number of people who called themselves friends and promised to keep in touch and those who actually do. We need to say that we certainly hope they will be the exception to the rule, but that in the meantime, it is too painful for the individual to risk going through another rejection. It is much better to be accurate and genuine about the status of the relationship today. You are not a friend. You are a good Supporter who has a deep caring for this person right now. There are no promises for the future in that role. There is only an achievable measure for the work that you have come to do today: care deeply for this person as you support her so that every moment counts to make a positive difference in her life.

It is not a shortcoming in a Supporter if she does not become a friend. Not providing good support is a shortcoming. There is no expectation for friendship. If it comes, we will only know later on and it is another thing altogether.

What is so wrong with calling a support relationship a friendship? There are several important problems with this. First of all, it causes a lot of pain to the individual. There is immense pain in rejection and abandonment. Even if the Supporter is unable to keep in touch for very understandable reasons, for a person with few freely given relationships it feels like rejection.

Secondly, this confusion can distort what the Supporter and the person might do with their time. Friends do things together differently than a Supporter and the person they support. Friends often just hang out. It doesn't much matter what they do with their time as long as they are together. They don't need to pay attention to other valued roles, this is one. They don't need to worry about being too much in community spaces, they are already enjoying relationship. This is true. We see Supporters hanging out with people at home, inviting the supported person to their own homes for no particular reason, or going to movies, going for a drive, mall walking and doing other things where other relationships are not inclined to enter. These relationships are friendly and isolating. When the Supporter leaves, there is only a void.

On the other hand, Supporters need to pay careful attention to the kinds of roles that the person is holding, the kinds of community settings in which they are present, and the kinds of other people they might encounter. Since the relationship with the Supporter is not the focal relationship, all of the Supporter's attention must be given for designing a context for new relationship to blossom (see Chapter 7). So if the Supporter believes that *they* are the friend, they will stop putting their whole attention toward setting the stage for friendships to occur.

A third reason to end this confusion between Supporter and friend is that it gives a false message that one role is more important than the other. The fact is that the person with a disability requires some degree of thoughtful, conscientious, reliable support in their life. The person also requires friends. These two are not interchangeable although sometimes they may overlap. Occasionally, a person might be able to receive all of their required support from friends, but this is the exception. For the most part a unique partnership is required for the person to fully be alive and part of her community. Denying one third of this partnership limits the possibilities for the person.

This is something which I have come to feel deeply about over time. Some families tell me that they have experienced the exception and a one-time Supporter is now a friend. Some Supporters themselves tell me they are the exception. They have moved on to friendship with people they once supported. I, myself, am an exception. I have an enduring personal commitment to two people whom I have come to love dearly. Our family has helped Joe to move closer to us so that we can see him more often and we have met with him in our home or his once or twice a week for the past 15 years. I have known Beatrice for 21 years and she is a firm part of our lives, our holiday traditions and birthday celebrations. I first met each of these people when I was paid to support them in the early 1980's.

I know from Beatrice's point of view that I am the exception. At the beginning of our support relationship, we spent some time counting up the number of support workers she had ever had in her life. At that point, we counted 19 different support people. She believes that most of them left on very good terms with her, and that about half of them promised to keep in touch. When I ended our support relationship, after supporting her for more than six years, I did not promise to keep in touch with her. I did not promise friendship. I did invite her to breakfast the week after I left, and the week after that, and the next week again and so on for a year. Slowly we began phone calls back and forth to each other, held a few celebrations together and grew a real friendship together. Today, she is 'Aunt Beatrice' to our children and a frequent friend in our home.

I understand that friendship will sometimes happen and we should be thrilled when it does. But my experience tells me it is the exception rather than the rule. And when it is the exception, it will happen after the paid relationship ends. We need to work with the strategies where we have some hope of influencing the outcome. I think that we have a great degree of control over finding and choosing good Supporters. We have a great deal of influence over setting the stage so that love is invited to grow. And we have little control at all over whether or not in the fullness of time the mystery of friendship will occur.

Let us spend our best efforts on finding good people, providing excellent orientation so that they will become good Supporters, and hoping that we are also able to invite that spark of respect and joy to deepen the work in the time the Supporter is with the person. One or two over time may become friends. That is a gift and cannot be gained by our efforts to ensure good support right now.

Good support is all about designing opportunities for friendships to develop. It is about getting paid to build the opportunities. It is not about being paid to be the friend.

Perhaps there is a hidden gift in this dilemma. Perhaps in learning to see love and work with love in our day-to-day spaces, we will bring meaning and depth to our own contributions. If we can find moments to love without needing to attach a promise for friendship forevermore, how freely might we then give of ourselves.

The Varied Faces of Support

Caroline Ann refuses to commit to support on a certain time or day without a specific reason for that Supporter to be there. Brenda is more relaxed and easygoing when she is spending time with her next-door neighbour, Hilda, when she spends a morning with her sister-in-law, Barb, or when she has a visit from a neighbour. At times she feels fed up with a Supporter and tells them to leave (they do). John puts up with some formal support in order to put together some balanced meals every week, but he does not like to hang out with a support person in situations where it is fairly clear that he is being helped in some way. When pushed into these kinds of situations he will just run away until he gets time on his own. In these ways, people are telling us that we need to find ways to offer support that feel genuine, natural, practical and balanced. They do not want to hang out with Supporters who do not want to be there. They do not want to feel the unequal power balance of someone always doing for them. They do not want a Supporter just to turn up and hang out for no particular reason. The hanging out they do, they prefer to do with neighbours, family and friends.

This was not hard for us to figure out for Caroline Ann or John. In many areas, the support required could well be done in another way. For them, the challenge continues to be finding Supporters who are willing and able to work very few hours on a very flexible basis. Support that does not feel like support, I call it.

For Brenda, it is more difficult to figure out support in ways that feel right to her. One thing that has helped is to differentiate between support people who offer in-home support, and those who help her explore and hold on to roles in the community. This has led to a larger number of Supporters working in a given week, but she seems to deal with the variety very well. In addition, each time a new person arrives, Brenda knows that this means a change of pace, plan or activity. If she does not much like what she is doing, then this can change before too long. In the same way, if she tells a Supporter to leave, it is not too long before another person can see if they can spend a different kind of time together. We also try to make sure that Brenda has time every day and on weekends where she is with family or friends, which to her feels very different than support. Eventually, we think that we will figure out a way for Brenda to call on people for support rather than people arriving to offer it. We think that this latter support often feels imposed to Brenda, even when it is not so intended.

Rob, Jon and Tiffany require knowledgeable caring people to be around them at all times. This does not mean, however, that they do not express the same desire for natural, genuine support that does not feel imposed without their consent. However, their ways of expressing this are more subtle, and therefore we must listen more carefully. Their families and circles know that they are much more vulnerable to abuse and neglect because of their speech is so limited. Tiffany has gone through one long period of extreme upset that brought Linda to lead Tiffany's Supporters back to the very basics of listening to and supporting Tiffany. Linda and the Supporters (and indeed the whole circle) re-discovered that Tiffany prefers to be told what will be happening a few moments in advance of the actual event. She likes to be offered options, involved in conversations when she is in the room, and allowed ample time to listen to her own music. The importance of these small things can be forgotten in a busy day filled with other priorities. Tiffany has let us know, however, that these are some of her priorities.

Harriet, Rob's mother, knows that Rob needs and appreciates some opportunity to walk along the halls and lobbies of his Rougemount home without a support person right beside him all of the time. He loves the freedom of this movement, as well as the encounters with the neighbours he may meet—uninhibited one-to-one contact. One of the joys of his friendship with Susie was the time spent on his own with her, while the Supporter was in another part of the house.

We need to be always listening and watching for ways to offer support that allow the person to feel like a full and participating member of their family or community. We need to figure out the least amount of support for the maximum benefit.

From the Supporters' Point of View

It is helpful for families and others to be aware of the complexities of the support role from the Supporter's point of view as well. Both short and longer term Supporters are clear on the drawbacks and hurdles in taking on support work. Monetary issues are important. The pay is relatively low, especially for those with degrees or certificates that would qualify them to work within the school system or for local associations. Most families can only afford to offer contract work, rather than full employment with benefits. This is especially difficult for Supporters who are sole income earners for their family. This carries an expectation that Supporters will report and pay their own Canada Pension Plan earnings. When this is not done, Supporters will be penalized in their senior years.

Most positions with the families of Deohaeko are part-time positions. Supporters who need full-time jobs in order to manage family finances need to take on other work. From personal experiences over the years and our basic principles, we do not share Supporters, so this other work must be sought outside of our family group. We understand the strain that this puts on Supporters, but at the same time, we are aware that this decision has been a wise course of action for us over the years. This decision has ensured that our sons and daughters are seen as unique individuals, rather than as part of a 'caseload'. As well, we have eliminated this chance for dissension within our family group. We can empathize with each other over problems without needing to judge that family's supervision against our own for the same Supporter. We can give each other advice and support. The price that we have to pay is that some Supporters are unhappy that they must look for more work elsewhere.

We also know that on top of the above challenges for Supporters, the work itself is not easy. Family demands are often necessarily high, and Supporters require a large number of skills in order to do well. The work demands a high degree of consciousness and a readiness to take initiative and accept responsibility. Sometimes family tensions make it a difficult environment within which to work. Many Supporters come to family support work because they see someone else doing it in the community and the work looks light-hearted and easy. In fact, there are many layers to this work. It can be deeply satisfying, but it is rarely easy.

Other than the challenges of finding good Supporters and providing a good orientation, there are a few issues that arise for families. As I have said before, when things are working well, there is nothing like a good Supporter. These are some of those other times.

Jon's Story: Whose Work Is It?

Through Jon, among others, we have learned some important things about the strong link between Supporter motivation and recognizing or building great opportunities for and with a person.

For a couple of years, Jon went through a lot of Supporters. The turnover was unending and exhausting for his parents and those of us who tried to recruit new people time after time. We could only imagine what this period of time was like for Jon.

One of the things to suffer during this period of endless change, was the rhythm and predictability of Jon's week. Through a number of means, despite the turmoil, we had managed to piece together quite a list of roles and activities that attracted Jon, where he had some talent, and which would bring meaning to his weeks. People thought about this individually, chatted about ideas during circle meetings and even came together in a larger gathering of over twenty family members, friends, old teachers, and neighbours.

Over this time, we thought of ways to expand and broaden his shredding business, *J.B. Shredding*. This would include developing his interest in photography and painting, exploring his attraction with the Internet, taking advantage of his interest in wandering around the community, selling or offering his shredding by-products to pet-related companies, and more.

When we look back over time, an interesting pattern emerges. During the time that an energetic, organized woman spent time with him, Jon's business entered into a flurry of great, upscale marketing. They designed and produced bright, attractive colour brochures. They came up with a marketing plan, complete with a marketing 'pitch' for new customers. They maintained the two customers that Jon had at the time.

When Jon was supported by a young woman who was also an artist, a small card-making endeavour was started. Jon began to make and offer birthday and other greeting cards to his friends and neighbours. He would make them on demand, and was paid for his work.

When Jon spent time with a warm, motherly type who was very supportive of his Catholic faith, he began to attend the meetings of the lively co-operative Rosary Group, bringing his cake and other goodies to potlucks and other functions.

An engaging young Supporter hung out at a video rental store with Jon for a long time, and managed to land him a twice weekly job there. Jon was in his idea of heaven—videos galore. His job was to check and rewind returning tapes, and he received (oh, joy!) free rentals for his work.

As Jon spent time with a computer-literate Supporter, he began to develop binders full of his favourite topics—scary Halloween haunted houses, Florida, undersea sites and adventures.

All of these roles and activities held great meaning for Jon. He enjoys being a small business owner and making a modest income. He loves to spend part of his time shredding paper. He likes to make cards and offer them to others who clearly enjoy his work. He loves videos and felt good about a job for which he so clearly had the skills. He is a believer and finds satisfaction in his spiritual life, and a sense of belonging in sharing that with others. He likes to be in charge of printing up pages and pages on his favourite topics.

The downside of these endeavours was that each new Supporter was not successful at supporting or furthering the endeavours of her predecessor. This meant that when the energetic young business-minded woman went on maternity leave, the next person in line did not follow up with the marketing plan. The small card-making endeavour ended when that Supporter went on to take up a more full-time art career. Being participant in the Rosary Group was, for a long time, reliant upon one Supporter (now happily seconded by several neighbours who know Jon well). Jon's job at the video store ended when the Supporter leaving coincided with new management at the store. Surfing the net is reserved for the one person who has the best computer skills.

We have come to understand that this is not simply a case of poor information exchange, or poor supervision and guidance of new Supporters, or intentional subordination. In many respects, we did make sure that adequate information and guidance was available to the new person. We often gave them small, achievable tasks and asked them to let us know how things were going. But, we encountered all kinds of believable and unavoidable hitches. New customers did not seem attracted by *J.B. Shredding's* marketing scheme. The new management at the video store did not seem to value Jon's contribution or click with his personality like the old one had. Jon did not seem to want to make cards with other Supporters. Jon seemed to do some 'slotting' of certain Supporters for certain roles, as well. He came to prefer to work on the Internet with one person, etc.

What we see is that all of Jon's roles and activities in his week are uniquely and intricately linked to a number of factors. Success is linked to three things: his relationship with the Supporter, the Supporter's affinity for that particular role or activity (affinity being a rough combination of the right skills, an interest in that area, the right energy match, enough of a vision for what that role could be to trouble shoot problems as they come up), and the Supporter's motivation to work toward high expectations of Jon, the role in the community, and herself.

This is crucial to understanding why some people experience such instability in the roles and activities which describe their lives. As long as the Supporter plays such a vital role in determining what Jon does with his time, how he spends his time will vary as often as his support does. The best way to help Jon enjoy regular, predictable weeks is to recruit Supporters who value his work, have an affinity for that kind of role and understand the importance of a consistent role for Jon over time. The only other ways to build in consistency is when a significant piece of the support for Jon in some roles comes from someone outside of the formal, paid support role.

While this is now recognized, it is proving itself very difficult to work within. Jon is a young man who uses a beautiful and unique way to communicate with others. People can and do learn his complex system over time, but this requires interest, energy and enough time away from other tasks to do so. Jon also has an inquisitive and often mischievous nature, and therefore requires gentle re-direction and assistance to remain in his own areas at work. The way that we work is to believe that the right job is out there for Jon—one where his natural tendencies will be welcomed and easily supported by those at hand. It seems difficult to build natural supports into the work place, given these dynamics, so we are still reliant on finding Supporters with affinity for the work and reliable for Jon. In the meantime, at least, we better understand that the ever-changing profile of Jon's weeks is much less due to deficiencies on his part than lacks and deficiencies on our own.

We also understand that Jon is particularly vulnerable to this phenomenon because he has a good deal of paid support in his life. It is less of an issue with people who require less support, or when support can be shared easily with on-site community people.

Using Local Experts

We have had some good success with helping people develop skills and passions through Supporters who are first and foremost experts in another area altogether. For example, it took an artist, Diane, to bring out Tiffany's interest in painting and colour. Through this and other experiences we have found some benefits to working with Supporters who are 'experts'. One, they only need to learn about the person they are to support, and not, as with other Supporters, also about the content of the role or activity in which the person is to engage. They know the content of their particular area of expertise already so much better than we do, and they can concentrate on getting to know the individual.

Two, we do not have to worry about whether or not the activity or role is one of interest to this Supporter. They have already demonstrated their interest and love for this area of life. When Donna went to look for a doula to help her after Matthew's birth, she did not have to worry about whether Erin was interested in babies and children. Her choice of work as a doula already proved her commitment in this regard.

Three, Supporters who are local experts already know all of the connections that can take us weeks of internet search and telephone calls to achieve. Diane knew all of the art groups in Durham Region and Scarborough and was able to help Tiffany connect to the group that would suit her best.

Four, Supporters who are expert in a given field already know the next steps to take and can guide the individual (and sometimes the circle) in figuring the best alternatives. Erin helped Donna with lactation groups, vaccination schedules and recognizing developmental milestones. For the rest of us in Donna's circle, each of these would have taken extensive research.

Five, Supporters who are experts in a given area often hold very high standards in these areas, and also hold high expectations that people will be able to meet these standards. One of Brenda's Supporters who was an environmentalist assisted Brenda to undertake an extensive set of water quality experiments on a regular basis as her contribution to her park site project. Had a less qualified Supporter been asked to make this decision, many of us would have accepted the answer that Brenda would not be able to assist in such complex lab work.

Experts are not always available or interested in support work, but when they are there are decided advantages.

Not Comprehending the Support Role

When a Supporter does not understand their support role very well, the impact is real and sudden. I describe above what may happen when a Supporter believes they are a friend. The impact also has real and unfortunate consequences when a Supporter does not support the individual well to explore and hold valued roles in their community. The least of what happens in these situations is that the individual does not take up an enhancing social role that might bring a number of good things (a chance to contribute new relationships) to their life. In some instances, though, people's current positive roles flounder or vanish when support is not good. This often happens during the transition between one Supporter and the next. But sometimes this happens because the Supporter is not (yet) able to provide good support. The person loses a job because the support was not there. The person misses the chance to sign up for another art class because the Supporter missed the date. Sometimes this is due to poor time management skills of the Supporter, poor understanding of their support roles, or poor motivation stemming from an inability to see the inherent worth of the individual.

At times, Brenda has only managed to hold on to her valued social role of environmental steward by her fingertips. Even though her own interest has never waned, and though Supporters around her have agreed that this was an important role for her to maintain, there was a period of time when she did not seem to be getting to the site. Supporters cited car problems, poor bus schedules, poor weather, poor motivation on Brenda's part when asked if she wanted to go, arriving at work with the wrong shoes, and poor time management. And yet when Brenda's mother, Margaret from our board, or I pitched in to help her hang on to this role, Brenda' interest and motivation was always high.

This is a strong reminder to us about the extent to which the quality of the days and weeks of the person can be dictated by the energy, interests, and personal qualities of the Supporter. We have found that when the Supporter is not able to summon the interest about a certain role or event that we believe the individual finds meaningful, it will rarely take place, and if it does the experience will be mediocre in quality and not continue. In theory, it is part of the job for the Supporter to follow the interests of the person. In reality, much more often, it is a Supporter's excitement and interest that leads the person. This is not a bad thing if you are looking to exploring new areas. However, if you happen to want to pursue an interest that the Supporter does not share, this is a problem.

Who's in Control?

In the same way, a Supporter can have great power and control over many aspects of the person's life. When we ask ourselves what are the basic ingredients to the essence of home, most of us would respond with such things as privacy, security and having control over who enters, being king within your own castle, and not having to always be at your best. Yet, the moment that people in a support role enter into the homes of our family member on a regular basis, something happens to that home base of control. Usually, once a schedule (however flexible) has been set up, the Supporter enters the home regardless of whether the person really wants them there or not at that time. The Supporter knows all kinds of intimate details about the person and how they run their home and their life. Many points of these details are then communicated back to family members and others. People may be given options about many things in their home, but these are very often contingent upon how the Supporter is feeling that day, whether or not they have a car, whether they have enough time or money to do what is chosen, and whether or not the parent feels that such is a worthy choice.

To counteract some of these issues we try to put a number of things in place. For one, the imbalance of power is raised during orientation and often during discussions with Supporters. Good Supporters work hard to ensure a better balance of power.

We ensure that people are involved in choosing their own new Supporters in ways that are meaningful for them. Some people sit in on the interview. Some people spend some time with the candidate on their own before a final decision is made. Some people have the candidate work for a short while several times and tell us with their actions how they feel about the new Supporter.

We try to make sure that when Brenda asks—or tells—a Supporter to leave, that she does so. We emphasize that listening to Brenda in these circumstances is more important than filling in the scheduled hours. We try to make sure that schedules change often to suit the individual and we let Supporters know to expect this to happen.

Personal Integrity

We have encountered thankfully few problems involving the personal integrity of Supporters, but even these few have made us vigilant. These have included fraud and forgery, and theft. Some incidents are at a low level such that the Supporter would not even truly consider them to be crimes. For us, one example was using one's own air miles card to collect points at the grocery check out rather than the one owned by the supported person. Others include slipping one or two grocery items for oneself into the cart, going out for meals and submitting tabs that are clearly beyond the individual's budget and lifestyle, and 'volunteering' in a crisis and then billing for every single hour. We've had a couple of instances of Supporters misappropriating bank funds. This has led families to put better checking-up systems in place to protect the meagre accounts of their family member.

Poor support, inability to follow the interests of the person, and issues of integrity are all important issues for families. We deal with them in a number of ways. We are aware of the impact of each factor on the lives of the people who receive support. Talking among ourselves and sharing stories of struggle keep our awareness high. So, we remind each other of the limits of support, of what can happen when a Supporter is unable to fill her role, of energy and interest dilemmas, and of keeping an eye on places where the individual is especially vulnerable to being taken advantage of. Secondly we believe that providing a good and thorough orientation allows families and others to foresee well in advance where the particular struggles for any given Supporter might be. Thirdly, we just keep on trying to find new and better ways to surround individuals with good, caring and effective support. Despite the struggles and the failures, this alternative remains a much better option than its service alternatives.

The Basics Endure

Eight years ago, I wrote a summary of some practical things that we had learned about Supporters and how best to fold them into our lives. We had a short list:

- One Supporter, one person at a time (e.g., no group support involving more than one person with a disability and one Supporter).
- One Supporter, one family (no sharing Supporters).
- No recruiting or hiring from within the Rougemount Co-operative membership.
- There are two kinds of Supporters: Homemakers and Facilitators.
- Use paid support primarily for in one's home or for outside of the co-operative (e.g., try to use natural supports as much as possible within the co-operative).

I am struck by the extent to which this list is just as valid today as it was eight and more years ago. However, part of what we know about our work is that the basics do not change very much. In order for things to work well, the hard part is that we must continually go back to the beginning again whenever new Supporters come on board.

Coordinators

A coordinator (often referred to as a facilitator in some areas) can be any paid person who provides one or a number of non-direct support roles to the family or family group. For some, this is a person who has some functions for the family group as a whole (proposal-writing, preparing funding accountability forms, bringing common concerns and experiences to the whole group, general recruitment). She then may have other roles in which she supports the individual families (helping individual families apply the group's general philosophy and principles in practical situations, assistance in interviewing, helping maintain circles, help to orient and guide Supporters, etc.).

In other situations, the coordinator may work for one family and simply have a few non-direct support duties in addition to her direct support roles. She may be asked to coordinate the schedule of paid and natural support, to handle budget and finances for the individual (with appropriate accountability), or to be the person with whom the family enters into discussion about what the supported person does with their time, etc.

We have used a coordinator model from the very beginning of our funding, ten years ago. There has been much interest in how we manage, use and think about this position from other families and family groups since we have worked in this way for a significant period of time. Therefore, I am going to devote some time and attention now to providing a bit of an overview of my role—my tasks and the approach I take—with Deohaeko Support Network. Our coordinator model follows the first example above, where I have both roles with the family group as a whole, and then other roles with the particular families.

We know that this is a key position for families and family groups like ours. Our coordinator helps each family individually, and the group collectively, map out and hold a vision for the longer term, while making sure that what happens now is sound and thriving. For us, one part-time coordinator for our seven families is extremely important to helping us build circles of support, establish connections in the community for our sons and daughters, find and orient new Supporters, and plan a solid foundation for the future. In our experience the degree of helpfulness and significant support from the coordinator happens when there is a low coordinator to family ratio. Currently, our ratio of seven families (where age and health issues are prevalent) to one 20-hour per week coordinator (with experience) is tight, but usually sufficient.

Our experience tells us that a facilitator or coordinator must be hired by and work for the family or family group—

that is, unencumbered by either agency or government association. This independent nature of the coordinator will ensure that the family remains in control of the priorities, goals, and life directions together with their family member. It is important to understand the ongoing mutual nature of this relationship. The family constantly teaches the facilitator and keeps them grounded. The facilitator constantly offers ideas and alternatives that are easier to see at an arm's length.

The coordinator is also instrumental in enabling our families to deal immediately and effectively with times of transition and change.

In the experience of the families of Deohaeko, the unique relationship that has developed between family members and their coordinator, as well as the highly satisfying nature of the work, has led to me, as coordinator, remaining together for well over ten years at this point.

SRV Around the Kitchen Table

I came to the families with my own values and beliefs from the very beginning. Long before I met with the families of Deohaeko, I had encountered the ideas and the teachings of Wolf Wolfensberger. I studied, listened, read and came to an appreciation of his thoughts on devaluation, people with disabilities, and the social role valorization framework that would give some positive direction to my work.

In my role as coordinator, together with families, we have taken much time to talk about why and how things would be done. I have come to more fully appreciate the truth within the SRV framework, and feel that a large part of my role is to share this understanding with families. Based on this view of the world and society's impact on people with disabilities, I have clear opinions on how society views people with disabilities, and what we can do to safeguard their lives and support them to take their full place in community. This means that I do not have an 'anything goes' approach to the ideas and plans of families. I believe that some approaches are more helpful than others; some ideas are not as benign as we might think; some ideas will result in people being seen in very negative and hurtful ways. I know and believe that the families of Deohaeko love their sons and daughters deeply, and want what is best for their lives. The SRV framework and my own personal values can offer them some ways of deepening their ideas and plans so they can ensure the lives of their sons and daughters.

I often call this part of my work, 'SRV around the kitchen table' since so much of the sharing and deepening of the concepts is done in small, informal discussions within people's living rooms and kitchens. I have learned to re-work and re-word many of the ideas into pieces that can be easily understood in a short timeframe and by people (families, circle members, Supporters, neighbours, friends) with very diverse schooling and background. I have come to understand that sharing these ideas is a further safeguard to the lives of the individuals we think about. It is also a way to support families and their allies to be strong in their support of their family member. There are many strands of 'SRV around the kitchen table' woven into many of my coordinator roles.

'Holding' the Vision with the Family

A large part of my role is to know the individual and the family well enough to be able to help them all articulate the vision that they hold of a good life for their family member. This does not happen quickly, but rather is an unfolding process that happens over a number of years. Listening to the individual is just as important a piece as listening to the family. Over time, I begin to more fully understand where their dreams and goals lie in terms of home, work/community contribution, relationships, leisure, spirituality, personal learning, lifelong achievements, health and well being, and more. I also begin to understand which parts of this vision are still unfolding as the individual is learning about all that life has to offer, and which parts are already firmly set. For Rob, Jon and Tiffany I have helped to put this vision in writing. I am in the process of doing so with John and Brenda. I may yet do so with the others.

Part of the coming to understand the vision, is that I then become one of the people who 'hold' the vision in the person's life. Within our circles, we talk about 'holding' in a reverent, non-controlling sense of accompanying people who carry a responsibility that might be better shared. In my experience, not many people in anyone's network have the time or the privilege to sit long enough with a family to truly hear their vision for and with their family member. This understanding of the full vision includes the cohesive picture of: an understanding of the significant events and stories of the individual and family's past, actively knowing, gathering, asking for details, and acting on important parts of the present to ensure a good life now, and imagining a positive future. During my ten years with these families, I believe that I have done so with a number of families. With that immense privilege comes the responsibility to hold the vision along with them. My responsibility is to be one of the people who know this big picture and am committed to share it with others and keep things on track by safeguarding the integrity of the vision and helping the family pass it along to others who will either honour it, work within it (Supporters), or begin to share and keep it safe.

Some of my most recent work is figuring out with families how to pass this vision on to the next generation who will be entrusted to ensure that the disabled family member live a good life after the parents' participation decreases or ends.

Safeguarding Valued Roles; Protecting Vulnerabilities

Roles are an important way for other community members to understand and value people with disabilities. Holding typical, valued, and recognizable social roles makes it more likely that community members will form relationships that are mutually enriching. It takes hard work and focus for people with disabilities to take on some of the life-defining social roles that most of us take for granted. At the same time, the same social forces place stereotyping negative roles on people and make them vulnerable to abuse and even violence. My understanding of these social dynamics, together with my deep care for the individuals that I have come to know, leads me to understand that one of my important tasks is to safeguard the current positive social roles that people hold.

I understand that the family roles that people have are vitally important to people's well being. I try to find ways to uphold and support efforts to strengthen and fill these family roles in natural and positive ways. I know that family roles such as son or daughter are already held in very positive ways. Sibling roles may not be as strongly held and we need to find new ways to fill them. People are beginning to hold some new roles as aunt, cousin, and step-son, as well and these offer lots of scope for new directions. Within circles and smaller discussions, we try to find ways to move forward in these roles. Sometimes, I am there simply to remind people that these family roles are there and only need to be embraced in small, natural, and typical ways (i.e., birthday cards, Christmas gifts, telephone calls).

Many of the community roles that people hold right now have been acquired since my time with the families, and I am fully aware of the richness that they have added to people's lives. I spend some time helping to safeguard these roles through tough times. When there is a transition of Supporters, when there are other problems in the family, or when medical or emotional issues arise, these roles are often threatened. I try to help make sure that this is only a temporary situation, or to provide some other way of holding the role. Sometimes, I do this directly, and often I just keep tabs on who is doing this in the interim.

When Tiffany's baking business was in some distress, her small advisory group met and we discussed how much the roles of entrepreneur and baker had added to Tiffany's life. After much effort, we found ways to scale down the work of the business without closing down completely, and with the intention of starting it up again when the right conditions prevailed. In addition, we talked long and hard within the larger circle and in smaller groups about what kinds of roles Tiffany might begin to explore to compensate. Her current roles as young artist and Rouge Valley naturalist were then born, and have grown to add much to her life. Sometimes I am there to help safeguard a role; sometimes I am there to make sure new and strong roles are ready to be explored as replacements. It is not to say that these good things would not happen without my presence, but rather that it is *my role* and responsibility to keep Tiffany's positive roles at the forefront of our thoughts.

I know that powerful, positive roles are a protection against the vulnerabilities that people possess. Sometimes I use this knowledge to balance out a strong negative perception that people may hold about a person. When Brenda is upset or anxious, all of her neighbours are likely to hear her distress. We know that this may lead some people to fear Brenda or to perceive her as a threat or a menace. To compensate and to remind her neighbours of the other side of Brenda, we try to find ways for her to meet her neighbours under positive circumstances. When she is invited to Tiffany's apartment for a gathering or party which always involves many of her neighbours, Brenda is invariably happy, gregarious and good-natured. We know that her neighbours need many chances to see her in this light, so we strongly encourage her to accept such invitations. Elizabeth, her mother, Brenda and I have discussed at length the conditions under which she is most likely to attend the event. As much as possible we try to bring these conditions about.

In many other ways, I work to promote the valued roles that individuals hold, and to protect against their vulnerabilities. I talk to individual Supporters when I can and reinforce their understanding of these dynamics. I talk to neighbours at Rougemount and try to counter their negative perceptions with good information, while promoting their understanding of people's positive roles and contributions at the same time. I talk to colleagues in places of work and to staff in recreation facilities, filling out their ideas about the lives that people lead. I do most of this discussion in very casual and familiar ways. Often it is only I who thinks in terms of roles and dynamics. I chat in casual, familiar ways about people and their lives, much like two neighbours or friends who gather to talk about a friend or a new acquaintance. Information is exchanged in the telling of small stories. Lasting impressions are formed through the sense of the ordinary. It looks and usually feels very casual; it takes quite a bit of intentional forethought.

As a Resource to Accessing the Community Spaces

I help families, circle members and Supporters figure out how to find and assess good places and roles in the community. Sometimes this is done in small discussions with the family and the Supporter, and sometimes within the circle. I don't have many personal connections in and among the clubs and networks in our area, but I do have a good idea of how they are organized and where one might go for further information. I try to help the Supporter or family figure out what they are actually asking for. I know that effective asking is based on asking the question to which the other person is able to say YES. The individual is involved in these discussions as often as possible – most of them take place in their home.

Often we begin with an interest that the person has shown or that the Supporter feels is worth exploring. I help to figure out all of the potential roles that people hold who share this interest, and then we work on all of the possible activities that are undertaken in these roles. Chapter 7 explores this process in more detail. It is an effective way to discover the many ways in which one might engage with their community.

Depending upon my time, the current skills and understanding of the Supporter, and the situation in general, I may offer to help with initial fact finding or contacts. There are several more steps outlined in Chapter 7 that may lead to a person exploring or holding a new role and engaging in new activities in their community. I may speak to Supporters as they work their way through this process, I may do a piece of it myself, or I may just be sought out as problems and difficulties arise. I do much of my own reading and following the events in our community, and I often pass along information about new groups, open houses and other opportunities for engagement.

Part of my role during this whole process is to model, teach and remind us all about the principles of social role valorization. I try to ensure that the roles sought are typical and valued, that the community settings frequented are valued in the community, that the activities enhance people's competencies and image, and that people can be reliably present on a intense basis. I try to find ways to remind Supporters that relationship building is key to their role and that must be vigilant in their efforts to invite, encourage and welcome people who are drawn to the person they support.

Helping With Orientation

I help families with different parts of the orientation process. For Donna and Brenda I am very involved in the entire process. For Tiffany and Jon, I often spend individual time with new Supporters talking about social roles, their roles and the principles behind our approach to support. For some of the others I do a small piece, or a one-time discussion. When trouble arises, I often work with the family to help the Supporter figure out the next steps. I am often involved in an ongoing dialogue with individuals, Supporters, and family members to deepen their understanding of the way in which we approach building a community of which this person is an integral part.

Promotion of Neighbourliness at Rougemount

I am at Rougemount at least three or four times every week and I make time for talking with neighbours about everyday things as often as possible. In this way, I try to keep abreast of the kind of information that I would want to know if I was living in that community. I try to bring this information back to the people that we support.

Quite often the information is familiar to them but a Supporter might not think through the implications. When it was announced that all of the locks were being changed on all of the unit doors, neither Brenda nor her Supporter at first understood how this might affect them. When I found out that changing the locks would mean men coming to hammer away at her door that was not broken, we knew that this would be difficult for Brenda to understand. We also realized the difficulty that having a new key would pose for Brenda. An everyday occurrence for most co-operative members (indeed also for the Supporter) was a situation that needed to be well worked out for Brenda.

Sometimes a person knows about the information but they are not sure what to do with it. When Marje was sick at home, people did not know if they should bring her a bowl of soup, or leave her alone in peace and quiet. From talking to Marje, I could help people think through what a welcome gesture to Marje might be.

Sometimes the person has not heard the information, and upon hearing it, knows just what they want to do. When someone in the community has died or has a close family member who has died, Donna is always the first person to buy a card and go around to get neighbours to sign it. Sometimes I am there to give her that information. More often she is the one that tells me what is happening.

Often, the individual would need significant support to react to news of the co-operative in typical, neighbourly ways. This is where I sometime try to play a role too. One day, a woman was down in the office very upset because her glasses were broken and she couldn't make it to the optometrist by bus before her kids got home from school. I knew Tiffany was home that afternoon, and I knew that she was with a Supporter who had a car. I asked the woman to wait while I checked something out and confirmed that Tiffany could move her plans around a bit and go with her Supporter to take this woman to her optometrist. I told the woman that her neighbour in #110 would help her out. Now, clearly, I could have done the same thing myself. But I knew that Tiffany might well have taken this opportunity herself if her time was free, and since she was the neighbour in a community wanting to promote neighbourliness, she was the better option.

Many times these hallway conversations tell me wonderful stories about many people in the co-operative. Keith who has provided maintenance for the building came to tell me about the great relationship he was developing with Brenda. I had a chance to put some of the extra repairs he needed to do for her into the context of Brenda being one of the people for whom this building came to be. Extra repairs would always be needed and that was okay. I heard about Keith being there the day that Matthew fell and broke his tooth.

People also use informal opportunities in the hallways and lobby to let me know about their concerns, often at an early enough stage that we can do something practical and immediate to improve the situation. In this way, I have heard that Matthew went out without mittens on a snowy day, that Brenda was up at 11:00 in the lobby the night before, that Jon's Supporter was awfully terse with him on the elevator, and that Caroline Ann came up for tea during the thunder storm. Most of these situations are easily looked into and I can bring some practical information back to the neighbour in a short time. I could tell them that Matthew was going out to a parked car. I could let them know that another neighbour saw Brenda, walked her home and stayed for a cup of tea until Brenda seemed ready for bed. I could say that it was good for Caroline Ann to feel so comfortable with them that she would choose to go there with her fears about storms. More importantly, however, is my joy at people's concern and attention for their neighbours. I let them know that caring about others in this way is helpful and positive. And, in the situation with Jon's Supporter at the time, the information was very important for the family so that they could keep an eye open and ensure Jon's well-being. In my eyes, this is community working just fine.

Keeping Track

People laugh at me good naturedly for the fact that I am always on hand with paper and pen, taking notes, recording. It is partly my nature that I think best with a pen in my hand. But it is also one of the ways that I contribute to the families and the group as a whole. I keep track. I keep notes about decisions that we have made as a group, things to do, good ideas to try out, and commitments that we have made to each other. Sometimes, I am sure, this merely makes me annoying. But it is also a part of me helping to hold and convey the big picture. If I keep track of much trivia, then the families don't need to. It's there for all to see, and much of it is copied, but it is not their responsibility alone to keep track. I can play that role.

I also keep track of some things in bigger ways. I have helped at least three families articulate a written vision for and with their son or daughter. These have developed into full-scale binders of information that we call, "All about Tiffany." The majority of the information in the vision and in the binders come from the families themselves. It is full of their ideas about content, scope, details and strategies. My part has been to introduce a format, organize the content, and to write in ways that fully reflect the original intent, our basic principles and values, the integrity of the person, and the uniqueness of this family.

I keep track on the writing of documents like our philosophy statement. This document has come about as a result of hours and hours of discussion among family members. My task was to try and record the discussions and then to produce many drafts of a document that reflected the ideas of the families. Each draft was then edited and subjected to more discussions and changes. My role was indeed to keep track.

Trying Another Way

When things go wrong, as they often do, I spend time with people trying to figure out what happened and what to do next. To me, this is more than a brainstorming or trouble-shooting role. This is where I have to have the strength and the ability to go back to our core principles in the middle of chaos and calamity. The family is often in the eye of the storm, torn between seemingly impossible choices or alternatives. I have a measure of distance that I try to use to help me find balance and direction from the things that we believe in. We often cannot follow the paths of those who have gone before us, because we are walking new ground. But we can make sure that everything that we try is at least in the context of the principles that we have set for ourselves. Some of the questions I ask myself and the family are:

- What happens for typical people when they find themselves at this point in their lives? (see a doctor, talk to a friend, start again, let time heal.)
- This may not be good but are the alternatives worse? If yes, then hang on to this position and ask for more time.

Brenda went through a period of great emotional distress and anxiety about a year ago. Many of the people around her wanted to put her psychotropic drugs to "manage her behaviour". Her mother knew and I agreed this was not the answer for Brenda, and we feared that the sensitivity she showed to other medication might in fact cause these kinds of drugs to backfire, placing her farther and farther into the drugged world.

During many deep discussions, Elizabeth and I decided that we thought that Brenda was having fairly typical reactions to several things in her life. There had been a great turmoil of support over the past five months, with a number of Supporters leaving and that uncertainty was very hard to handle. Elizabeth had been very ill with a flu a couple of months before and had not seen Brenda very much at all. Brenda had reacted very strongly to her father's death years ago, and often talked about her fear of her mother dying. She must have been feeling that fear very strongly. We felt that Brenda might be experiencing symptoms of early menopause that showed up in family history.

We tried to put ourselves in Brenda's shoes, wondering what we might do if we found ourselves in a similar situation. It was clear that Brenda's emotional distress was acute much of the time and we did want to find a way to help her to feel better. We thought that for ourselves, being people not inclined to take medication for our ailments, we might consult a homeopathic or naturopathic doctor. And so, following the word-of-mouth advice from a colleague, Brenda came to meet Dr. Joe Kellerstein. Dr. Joe listened and asked questions and listened some more. He helped Elizabeth draw parallels between Brenda's showing of rage and that of her grandmother. He helped us to see aspects of learned behaviour in her patterns of anger. He gave Brenda a very low dose of remedy and then taught us to observe Brenda well. We learned to look for signs of upset and reasons for upset, changes in how she showed her anger and symptoms of other good things happening in her life.

Life is not perfect for Brenda and those who care for her. But nowadays when she has one upset, it no longer means that she will have a day full of upset. Upsets rarely interfere with the day's plans anymore. We continue to see moments of anxiety and anger, but we also see some new highs. Brenda likes to sit and focus on being read to from fairly complex chapter books. Brenda is producing some art that she feels proud of and happy to frame and give away. We look at Brenda and her emotional state. We understand that her upset and rage might come from a combination of factors. Some we have control over and some we do not. This has been a rocky road, fraught with contradictory advice from good people. Elizabeth, Brenda, the rest of her family and I have chosen a path that is not easy for many others to accept or believe in. However, it is a path that has honoured our principles. It is a valued choice that we would make for ourselves; it is not experimental any more than trying psychotropic drugs on a woman who has not had them is experimental. Brenda's uniqueness has been upheld—we know that she needs and demands to be supported in genuine ways and we strive for that. We have accepted a part of the responsibility for her anxiety and anger in acknowledging that the support for her is still imperfect.

Through this process I have also gained some insight into what helps me when I am with Brenda and she is upset. I apologize. I tell her that I am sorry. I am sorry that she is upset. I am sorry that I confused her in some way and I don't know what. I am sorry that I can't figure it out.

Then I am silent. And then she is okay again. I think in the space that we allowed ourselves to pull back from medical answers, I have found out some more about Brenda.

I think that Brenda will always be a person with a volatile nature. But her highs are much higher than her lows are low, and it is in her highs that you come to love her. On a day that I rushed in and said in passing that I had forgotten my lunch, she brought me an apple. It's my last one, she smiled. On a day of a very big upset, she sat down and made a remarkable replica of a flower in pastel. Makes me think of an artist's temperament. Brenda brings gifts for Matthew, gifts for Hilda, flowers for her Mom, and goodies for many people. How can we take the edge off her anger without taking the edge off her heart?

I don't know what the future will hold for Brenda in terms of effective ways to help her feel relaxed and calm. I only know that I will continue to move with Elizabeth, Brenda and other family members to choose ways that uphold our principles. These allow us to see Brenda as a unique individual; choose alternatives that typical, valued citizens would choose first; and recognize that at least part of the reasons for Brenda's anxiety lies with factors external to Brenda herself—worries about family health, support that does not feel right, and inconsistency in that support.

Helping With Recruitment

My role in helping families find people has changed quite a bit. Until about a year ago, I or someone in my position really took charge of the initial steps. I posted notices (drafted together with the family), received resumes, did telephone screenings of all resumes, and passed along vetted candidates to families where the request seemed to match the resume. I then went on to assist only occasionally with interviews, references and letters of offer. This always varied from family to family.

Over the past three or four years, we have tried in vain to hire a person to take on this concrete assistance to helping families find new Supporters. We believe that it is very hard to do this part of the job in isolation from really getting to know the individuals and their families. In the past year, I have had less time to devote to these tasks and families take on a bigger part of posting notices and looking for Supporters. At the same time, there are fewer places than before to post openings and expect a flood of resumes. Searching for Supporters is a less formal process than a year ago. As a result, more of our time is taken up in word-of-mouth recruitment. This means that resumes and telephone inquiries go directly to families as often as they come to me. The resume and telephone screening tasks are now shared more directly with the families.

Plan Board-Family Retreat Focus

As part of our annual renewal, all of the family board members go away on a one and a half-day retreat every November. We have carried on this tradition for ten years. My part in this event is to help the board plan a focus for the year's event, and then to implement some creative way to initiate discussion of the issue. Over the years, we have been fortunate enough to work with two coordinators (due to a small funded project) three or four times. These have resulted in dynamic, creative events. One year the board was kidnapped and forced into leisure pursuits of frivolous kinds. Another year, we created a whole game in order to re-create a scenario to help us choose the right kind of endowment fund to meet our needs. On my own, retreats may be less glitzy, but still provide creative ways for the families to talk about future plans, assess past successes, tell stories, and solve bigger problems.

Being With People

There are times when we are temporarily stymied. We can't find the support, or the role is not working out, or the people around just don't get it, and in the end the person is let down again. At these times, the single most important thing that I can do is to be with the person. This happens for some people more than with others, but often it is in the 'being there' that I can offer comfort, a practical hand, and the promise of my presence. These are hard times, but very personally, they are also good times. The reality of our situation stands beside me. I don't have an answer, but I may have an hour or so just to be. This is a very fulfilling part of my role, and often serves to renew me, stir up new ideas, or just feel right for the moment.

Funding and Budgeting Responsibilities

I keep track of funding proposals, which includes writing them together with the families, and producing reports as necessary. Not only is this an administrative load off families, but it ensures that our requests are made in a coherent fashion, based on the principles which we have all worked on together.

I work closely with the families to understand the nature of supports required for their families and to assess potential sources of funding (government, Trillium, crisis, foundations, other). Once this has been done, I write the funding proposals on my own and return to the family or the whole group, depending on the type of funding sought, for final edits and approval. Often, I establish the communication links with funders so that they have a consistent person to address questions and requests for information. However, all funding proposals and all formal communication are approved by the family or the group, and are sent under the appropriate family or group name. Once again, my role is to ensure the smooth and articulate flow of information, not to establish personal responsibility. In this way, I act much more in the role of funding consultant than executive director.

Our funding is received by the board as a whole in almost all situations. This, together with our hard-earned fundraising dollars, makes up our annual budget. Every spring, I draft the next fiscal year's working budget which the board goes over in detail, changes and finally approves. We have contracted with a very part-time administrator to manage our banking, write cheques on behalf of the board (but not the individual support dollar payments which are made directly by families to Supporters), and submit monthly budget statements to the board. My role throughout the year is to help the board understand the monthly statements.

I also keep track of the accountability formats for our transfer payment agency. This only means that I provide a global record of the fact that all dollars received went out to families every month; the families maintain their own records. Finally, I keep track of the details of our annualized support dollars from the provincial government and the expenses of our five year Trillium grant.

Other Issues for Coordinators

Refusing to Take Full Control

No matter what the role of the coordinator, a key lesson that we have learned is that this person should never take over full responsibility from a family or designated, unpaid circle member.

This means that even when the coordinator is asked, for example, to coordinate the schedule of paid support, the family should always be aware of changes and variations to the schedule. They should certainly be called if last minute arrangements have to be made due to inclement weather, Supporter illness, etc. In many cases, the family does know about these incidents simply because they are called in to be with their family member, as a sort of back up. However, a family member should know about all of these changes for several reasons. For one, it gives a clear message to paid Supporters that the essential difference between this person's home and an agency-controlled service setting is that a family member is in charge.

Secondly, it is more difficult for a Supporter to call in repeatedly to a family member to report car troubles, illness and sundry other reasons for being absent, than it is to another paid person. It is, therefore, another reminder that the Supporter role is vital, and that their absence for any but the most serious reasons has an impact on the whole family.

Thirdly, a family member must always have a full picture of the nature of the week that the disabled family member is experiencing. If the family does not hear about the three or four last-minute support changes as they are occurring, they might not understand the impact this must be having upon the supported person themselves. When they are current with changes as they occur, they can begin earlier to look for ways of increasing stability for their family member. It is not that a paid coordinator will not do so, but often for the coordinator if they are able to make an alternate arrangement so that support is provided, they will feel that they have done their job. This is not lack of empathy on the part of the coordinator. I have been in that position myself. However, sometimes back-up plans are very difficult to make and take many phone calls to arrange. After all that, it is hard to sit back and say that, "things must be done differently!" It may be difficult to additionally place themselves in the shoes of the supported person and figure out that what you have just done is piecemeal at best.

Wolf Wolfensberger in his book, *The Future of Children With Significant Impairments: What Parents Fear and Want, and What They and Others May Be Able To Do About It,* (2003) lays out clearly the problem with handing over responsibility for your family member to a system of paid services. He says that they often end up under a power equal to that of a parent, but without the love that a parent has for their child. He outlines how, time and again, this is a set up for violence and abuse. He calls this one of the universal laws of violence.

Now handing over full responsibility to a paid coordinator for taking care of support schedules may not seem like handing over responsibility to a paid service system, and maybe violence will not result. However, the true threat lies in the family assumption that *anyone or anything* can fully take over such functions without a controlling role for the family. If the coordinator fully takes it over and does it poorly, will a local service system that offers to coordinate regular support be the next choice? If the local service system has difficulty managing support and offers your family member a 'temporary' place in a group home would that become acceptable? If "the family remains in control" is the mantra of the support situation for your family member, these other scenarios will not be contemplated, and this particular risk of violence to your family will be reduced or eliminated.

This is not just the case for the scheduling of support. It is the same for all of the tasks that might be assigned to a coordinator. The wrong message is given when total responsibility for orientation of new people is given over to current paid people. This is a staffed model where Supporters are in charge of 'what is best'—even when they have only been around for a year or two in some situations. Family, or a designated person who has demonstrated their caring for and knowledge of the person over time, must remain in control of orientation. They may delegate portions of it to Supporters, but they must hold the whole of the orientation, for it is they who must ultimately assess the progress of the individual and their ability to provide good support.

When a coordinator takes over the whole of the recruitment-interviewing-hiring process, once again the individual and their support structure will suffer. Families need to be at the centre of this process as well. Of course, it is helpful and time-saving to ask a coordinator to draft a posting, distribute postings to agreed-upon sites, prepare good interview questions, and draft the family letter of contract offer. But family must find a place to position themselves early in the conversation. For us, once I have determined that the person's availability and basic skills seem to meet the current opening, I pass them along to the family for telephone conversation and to set up the details of the first interview. I may or may not be present for the interview. I assist in setting up the working interview, at which I am rarely present. I may return again for part of the orientation process, and when I draft the letter of offer for the family to edit and sign. In many respects, I maintain the flow and the pace of the hiring process, but I am not very visible and most Supporters are very clear for whom they are working by the end of this process.

My role is most often to be aware of and involved in the whole (the process, the picture, the funding proposal, the principles and philosophy) that the families have already agreed upon. I maintain the pace, remind about next steps or practical applications, and often (but not always) invite evaluation. But while I 'hold' much of the big picture, I refuse to do so alone. This is not mine, it does not belong to me. My role is to work alongside or to walk alongside, but it is not to move on alone.

Alone, I have no role to play. I cannot be responsible and committed for the vision on my own. I support but I cannot carry the lives of seven or more individuals and I am not rooted in the reality of a living family (within this group). Alone, I become a threat. In order to cope, I would have to develop abstract policies, schedules with guidelines, and rules on how things should be done. Alone, I would only serve to isolate. I would enter into a world we want to avoid—a world of paid coordinator, paid support, and disabled person at the core, family and friends on the outside. My responsibility is not to go there. The family responsibility is to not to let me.

I remain highly visible to the families, and often barely visible to many others. This duality is also important. Families must know what I am doing, and how I am doing it every step of the way. It is the only way that it can remain theirs. At the same time, our society most often views families—particularly families who have children with disabilities—as incompetent. Families are not incompetent. In fact, it is their very competence at a whole new set of tasks during a stressful time in life that have them juggling work loads and expectations that programs and corporate entities could never hope to accomplish!

This is one of the reasons, however, that it is important for me to reduce my visibility in more public spaces. I do not want others to misunderstand my presence and the hard work that I do as doing instead of the families. Others will presume my competence; they will not do so for the families. They will not see that I have my set of skills and families have theirs, and it is in our work together (and in our common heart) that we accomplish so much. Ways that I reduce my visibility include rarely, if ever, speaking on behalf of Deohaeko Support Network without the co-presence of a family member. We can then each speak from our own experience. In dealing with Supporters, I make sure that the family role is clear, even in the few times when they are not present. I try to write proposal submissions, and reports in such a way that any paid coordinator might be doing the writing, and I refer most often details and questions to family/board members.

A Second Coordinator

We have struggled to find a role for a second coordinator that works well. We have tried a second coordinator with a similar skill set. We found that we could much more easily find someone with either the family work skills or the administrative-money management skills, but not with both (with the exception of Alison MacArthur who was with us in this role from 1995-1998. We have tried several coordinators with only administrative kinds of skills, but have not been very successful in retaining them, possibly because the work became very isolated from the rest of what we do and the person ended up being quite on their own and not feeling part of anything. We have no office, no regular meeting times except monthly board meetings, and little down time to just build relations. This is a difficult work context for many people, especially since they have most likely built their administrative skills repertoire in an office setting. In between second coordinators, I would pick up the work until a new person could be found. I'm sure this has led to a reluctance to let go of things on my part.

Unique Characteristics of the Deohaeko Experience

There are a few elements that characterize the experience of the Deohaeko families working together with a family coordinator. First of all, as coordinator I have worked alongside the families of Deohaeko since their first small chunk of funding, over ten years ago. This long commitment has clearly had some benefits to us all. There has been time to develop a deep level of trust, which shows up at many times, but particularly when difficult decisions need to be made.

Secondly, I was present when we worked together to articulate common principles so that these are not a set of principles that the families have handed to me to follow, but rather a set of principles that I feel that I was a part of defining.

Thirdly, in part due to the length of time I have spent with the families of Deohaeko, and in part due to the mystery that surrounds all relationships, I have genuine relationships that are deeply embedded in caring and trust with all of the individuals who receive support. I would honestly say that most of the time the highlight of many of my days are moments spent with one or another of the individuals themselves. This lends a deep quality and a depth to the work that I do. It matters.

Fourthly, I have been there long enough to have tried many things, and I have a good understanding of what works and what does not work in very practical terms. Being in place for so long ensures that I do not have to repeat errors made in the early days of little experience. In many work situations, there is such turnover that errors made by a person in a new situation, occur on a frequent basis. I certainly continue to make my share of mistakes, but not the ones due to inexperience.

Finally, the stability of my work over time and within the relationships with the families has allowed me time for reflection, comparison and learning. I have had the benefit from staying with and understanding a set of circumstances quite deeply. Due to my own interests this has led me to writing—books, individual accounts, small stories, chapters in longer works, tools and strategies for our own and wider use. This happy correlation of the time and stability of the work, overlapping with my own growing abilities and skills has resulted in quite a bit of written materials, useful for both the present and for anyone in this role in the future.

Identifying Some of the Struggles

In the task of finding any coordinator for a family group or even for a single family, I think that the following considerations are essential.

It is important that I support the family group, offer advice and direction based on principle and experience, but do not take over. This does not mean that I support anything that comes forward. But it means that I have spent many, many hours in discussion with the group about the common values and principles that will guide us. Then when decisions are considered which go against these, I feel comfortable in pointing this out to the group. It helps that we are committed to consensus decision-making, so we work hard to ensure that we understand each other well before we go ahead.

The families and the coordinator must be very clear that the role of the coordinator in the future is not to replace the parent. I will assist in the building of a circle or in the strengthening of family bonds and understanding so that these groups can take on the broader roles that will be required in the future. Stability and commitment lie within family and friends; paid allies can and will be supportive and helpful, but not a governing agent.

Related to this point is the fact that this work can have periods of great intensity, especially since I am working with a group of families. But high intensity cannot be sustained. All situations of crisis need to be resolved fairly quickly, at least to the degree that the coordinator resumes a more supportive (rather than direct) role. This frees me up to return to other areas of my role which have been neglected during the crisis or to regain time with my own family. At the same time, this ensures that I do not become the main person in the event of a crisis. On my part-time status, I simply could not manage this role for all families. I can only help families to manage the struggles they are going through. The limits of my time are a curious but effective safeguard for the principle of family control.

In conclusion, I believe that the role of supportive allies is key to the well being and good support of individuals towards their dreams. However, they have been cast into a supportive role, not as the primary star, and that difference should never be forgotten. There is an Emmy award for best supporting actor, as there is for best actor. They have different roles and different functions, and they are judged, in the end, for their individual performances for the role at hand.

In the same way, as long as coordinators and Supporters are viewed as tools to be used well and wisely in order to work the soil, you can set your sites on a better garden. But when the tools and strategies are more prominent than the flowers and plants themselves, they will only diminish the beauty and the strength that lies about them.

Section 4
Over Wintering in Preparation for the Spring Ahead

Chapter 9: Safeguarding
Chapter 10: Dancing in the Garden of Life

This last section of the book includes two very different metaphors. On the one hand, a chapter on safeguarding makes reference to the cold, dark and often dangerous winter season. For gardeners, the trick is often in the preparing the garden to make it through the winter: over wintering. The real danger is in the killing frost. A typical frost can change a green and yellow fall garden into the brown and dry stalks of winter scenery. But the killing frost will get at the very roots of a plant and end all hopes of a spring recovery.

Providing effective safeguards for the things we value and for those we love is to prepare for the killing frost. Experience shows us that we need to prepare for troubles ahead. We need to recognize problems when they are still in their infant stages. We need to be able to discern between problems that will be merely uncomfortable and those that may effectively curb or halt our dreams.

On the other hand, the final chapter begins with a image of light and life. Dancing in the garden of life is an optimistic, metaphorical look at our achievements. It highlights the changes and growth around us that have taken place merely on account of our presence, our perseverance and our understanding. It is that moment in the glorious sunshine of a July morning when we are feeling that all troubles are temporarily at bay. It is that single instant understanding that for right now we are right where we want to be and doing what we want to be doing. We know that under analysis, things are not perfect and could be made better in many ways. But we take the moment for what it is. For the moment things are good.

Proper over wintering will ensure the likelihood of such July moments in the summer ahead.

Further into chapter, we look at the key underpinnings of a good future for and with our family members. But this only comes about as a result of having those instances of pure joy. The aftermath of pure joy is a deep desire to return to that place, to safeguard it so that it can be attained again and again.

We think that looking after the financial future and the relationship future for and together with our family members are two strong safeguards to make sure that such joy will be possible in all of our futures. There are challenges in putting both of these kinds of safeguards in place. We've built a firm foundation, we've helped to set and deepen many roots. We're ready for a typical winter or the winding down of life in ordinary ways. But all plans are not yet secure for the time of over wintering without parents, although we've managed that once already. The rest of that story will have to come at a later time.

We are not despairing, however, and we point out our sources of faith and hope. The final safeguard to ensure return to moments of joy and rightness, is our ability to communicate that joy with others in such a way that they too, will want to work tirelessly toward those moments for the whole community.

Chapter 9
Safeguarding

In a cold January in the early years of the new millennium, events in Durham Region made me acutely aware of some of the things we had taken for granted in doing our work. A highly supportive local association, led by a capable and visionary executive director with the ability to inspire and encourage many, many people had been swept away by a new reactionary board. It felt as if the whole political landscape that formed the backdrop of our work and our lives had been changed overnight. How we would proceed was uncertain. The only certainty was that the way of doing things based on support and encouragement from a friendly community partner with the advantages of size, power and a voice at the right tables was now changed. An era had passed, it seems, and one that we forgot to enjoy. At this vantage point, this new era felt a little cooler and our work felt a little lonelier. It turned my thoughts to the issues of safeguarding—keeping safe what is near and dear to our hearts.

Truth to tell, a chapter on safeguarding did not appear as a section foremost in my mind when I wrote the original table of contents for this book, or even as I honed it more thoroughly a little later on. Yet during this time of change, there I sat, reading through and revising many other sections trying to re-capture the optimism of my earlier work. I would sit and work through sections that fairly accurately captured our approach, thinking and actions; I found my innermost voice whispering "Yes but now what…." And I would stop and have grave worries of how we would approach our work over the coming months given this new state of affairs. I slowly came to realize that an additional section had to be added to this book.

When I began this chapter, with these events heavy on my mind, I thought this was a chapter about mistakes. I even wrote at first, that it was a little bit about closing the barn door after the horses had gone. I defended doing so by noting that there were still things of precious worth in the barn. It was as if I thought we should have known the events that we about to unfold. But I think now that I was naive in believing that we could have perfect vision and ability to see into the future and predict the exact moment and details of the action. I was also naïve in believing that even if that were so, that we would have any power to stop the events from taking place.

I think at this point, that this is not a story about learning from our failure, but it is a story of example and some degree of success. It is a difficult story to be a part of, but at the same time what we believed, what we valued and what we had put in place to safeguard—much of that worked.

It's not perfect, but then life rarely is. And there are certainly elements we can learn from this story about things that we might have done and didn't—or didn't do nearly well enough. It will serve as a reminder to ourselves as to the work that we must now do right away, and as advice to those who have embarked on journeys similar to our own. This is relevant only because our livelihood—our life and dreams of our strong, healthy communities that we ourselves want to be a part of and which include everyone—depends on this information and way of thinking.

From our position right now, I can identify a number of other important situations at different levels for the Deohaeko families that called for safeguarding. Some of these are stories worth telling for what they have taught us about the basics and importance of safeguarding what we hold dear. It's not that we could have prevented the threat from occurring in these stories, but how we met that threat, prepared for it (or not), and learned when we made mistakes. In examining these stories, I am drawn to think about more general strategies and approaches to safeguarding. In general, four answers come to mind when I ask, "What keeps us (and what we value) safe?"

Awareness

Awareness is knowing what you have and value, and knowing what keeps that safe and what will put that at risk. I see this as the first step in preparing an effective safeguard against the things that put these at risk.

I think that we have become more and more clear about what we as a group of families and citizens value and believe in. The details are set down in writing in our statement of philosophy (partly outlined in Chapter 2). We value the very lives of our family members who have a developmental disability as unique and contributing citizens in their communities. We value their presence, the places and people that welcome them, and the ways in which they contribute to our community. We know that it is mainly people (directly and indirectly) who keep them safe and who support them to be present, active, and able to make the most of opportunities around them. We know that what keeps them safe is what is better for our communities as a whole. We know that it is societal efforts towards conformity, perfection, and segregation of differences that threaten our family members and responsive communities most.

Vigilance

Vigilance is recognizing and understanding the first signs that what you value and love is being put at risk. The threats may come from people, from well-intentioned rules or laws, from actions that are not well intentioned but are launched out of fear or retribution.

The greatest risks to our family members and our vision of community can come in small incremental steps. These threats are, therefore, harder to see and take constant and careful vigilance to pick up in the early stages. The following are a range of stories about the ways that what we value may be put at risk.

Brenda had been pronounced environmental steward of her park site by Pickering City Council and was working in that role for about a year. I was talking to a coordinator of watershed project who was very enthusiastic about Brenda's work. She said that Brenda had inspired her to conceive of a whole new project, which would be to parcel up other park areas along the watershed and then call local associations looking for disabled people who could then be given stewardship titles like Brenda's. I was appalled. Brenda's hard work and claim to the environmental stewardship role had little to do with her disability and everything to do with her love of nature and dedication to this little park. The uniqueness of Brenda's contribution to her community was put at risk, as well as the importance of her role in the eyes of the watershed project.

Mary came to me one day with another story of a Supporter who needed time off while another one was still recovering from surgery, and a third one was dealing with family stresses. "Jon is always third" she said, "Supporters' families come first. Work, and not just this work, comes second. And Jon is third." This was Mary's articulation of the constant threat to the stability in Jon's life. She wasn't disagreeing with Supporters' order of priorities. She had simply learned to see the facts in front of her and understand that her son also needed people who would put him first in their lives.

We have told the story of Rob's journey from sharing his home with roommates in different ways, to exploring one-bedroom apartment options, to settling into a two-bedroom apartment with a Supporter who sleeps over. While this last situation is clearly the one that works best for Rob in terms of stability, predictability, and space issues, it is also the one that contradicted the co-operative's housing policy at the time. This policy was set by the Ministry and administered by the board of the co-operative and allocated a minimum of one person per bedroom. We knew this living situation would put Rob at some risk for being judged as 'over housed' and having to return to one of the earlier, unworkable living arrangements.

Tiffany was working her third year at the Rouge Valley Butterfly Garden when two events happened at the same time. On the one hand, she arrived one day to find another small garden beginning to be set up nearby—one that was childishly labelled with a girl's name. She was told that another woman with a disability was going to set up a garden nearby and the woman's support staff had decided that naming these gardens after their gardeners would be a nice touch. They offered to prepare a similar label for Tiffany. Once again, Tiffany's significant contribution to the Butterfly Project was at risk of being diminished, changed from an acknowledged contribution to a situation where Tiffany was the main beneficiary of the project's 'kindness'. At the same time, Tiffany was given a flyer by one of the Rouge Valley volunteers stating that Thursday was about to become Camp Day at centre's main building and Tiffany would be welcome to join other people with disabilities for a weekly day in nature. Once again the grave risk was that the uniqueness of Tiffany's interests and contributions would be well hidden under the overwhelming perception of her as a disabled person taking part in special, segregated and different events at the Rouge Valley.

At one point in the partnership between Deohaeko Support Network and the Rougemount Co-operative there was an opportunity to solidify and formalize the ongoing practice of having two Deohaeko board members (who were also founding members of the Rougemount Co-operative) sit on the Rougemount Board. However, this had always been the case, and just two years before there was a vote among the membership that this should continue. Deohaeko was acknowledged as the keeper of the flame of intentional community and the members were held in high esteem also for their considerable knowledge about how to work a board. The risk of this changing seemed remote to all of the members involved. When a period of dissent came to the co-operative community, the risk to this arrangement was not noted.

One summer evening as I was in touch with almost all of the individuals supported by Deohaeko, I slowly came to realize that each one of them was invited to a barbecue that night at the home of one of the Supporters. Most of the people did not know others from Deohaeko were attending and believed that they were attending a barbecue for the Supporter's family and neighbours. I felt uncomfortable with the segregated social event that had been arranged. My concern was less for the one-time event than it was for the Supporter's thinking behind planning such an event, and the message that would be given out to other Supporters who might be going along to accompany one of the guests. This was a threat to the ways in which the families of Deohaeko had imagined to use valuable Supporter time. It flew in the face of our understanding that people are safer and better off in fully inclusive community events, and that Supporters are our allies in planning inclusive events.

These are a sampling of the stories and situations that we face on an ongoing basis. What is most important is that we are clear on what we value from the start, we are vigilant and aware of when our ways are at risk. The next step is to be prepared for appropriate action.

Prepared for Action

Being prepared for appropriate action means knowing what to do when danger strikes and having a ready-to-go tool kit of strategies to put in place. These will include people to consult (friends, allies, circle members, lawyers, organizational consultants), sources of information and analysis that you can trust, the commitment to set aside time to think and talk with others when your priorities are threatened. This also involves anticipating the 'strike' and having a fallback position if things do not go your way. What might you have to give up? What will you give up in order to protect something else? What will you change because you are not prepared to take that loss? Having all of this prepared in advance means that you will be that much more ready and able to react in positive ways when necessary.

The stories outlined above each move on to a course of action that helps to demonstrate the kinds of actions and strategies that may be helpful to ward off, minimize or deal with a threat at hand.

When the watershed coordinator told me about her project to create environmental steward positions across the bay for other people with disabilities, I was in a good position to **talk to a contact that has some power to change the course of action**. The coordinator and I had come to know each other fairly well over the past year. We both felt good about our part in helping Brenda to achieve her current status. Based on our relationship and mutual respect we were able to have a conversation about what such a project would mean for Brenda. I was able to remind her that Brenda had come to her based on her interests and skills, not based on her limitations and disabilities. The stewardship *was* a good idea of ours, but because it called forth the interests and energy of a citizen who had time to give, and not because it gave a disabled person something to do. As we talked, she began to see the merits of setting up the stewardship project as a way to attract a variety of interested, nature-loving citizens—a project that would focus on people's positive attributes rather than their limitations. This threat to the value and image of Brenda's positive social role was warded off because I was able to talk to the right person at the right time (early on). The fact that we had a respectful working relationship together in the past was probably crucial in her being able to understand my concerns without being defensive.

When Mary came to the realization that Supporters would necessarily look after their families and their working lives, before Jon's, this was the beginning of **a clearer understanding of the threats** and need for other safeguards in Jon's life. The heightened awareness alone is the beginning of shaping a better plan for Jon. As life would have it, we have found no immediate solution to this situation, although some close family members are a part of the picture. Mary and Clive understand that for the time being they must have **a temporary plan**. It is only they who are able and willing to put Jon first. But knowing that they can currently not rely on anyone else has made life safer for Jon right now. They are not relying on any false assumptions. They are quite prepared to put Jon first right now, and begin the search and encouragement for those who will do so in the future.

When Rob moved into his current two-bedroom home, his family and the rest of the Deohaeko families began a deliberate process in order to safeguard his situation, as well as that of others. We began to **educate all prospective allies**. For us that meant going to the Rougemount board and explaining in detail how this arrangement worked the best for Rob. Members listened well, asked questions and ended up fully supporting Rob's home. Part of their support to Rob and his situation came about because Rob has always been very **present in the community**. So in some ways, they were able to hear Rob's story better because they already knew him as a fine, contributing member of their community. He was not a stranger asking for an exception, but a member reminding them of his uniqueness. Finally, we **prepared in writing** a clear and detailed account of the reasons that Rob would require this kind of apartment arrangement for his home. We have had occasion to use this with the board, put it on Rob's file at Rougemount and present it to the Ministry of Housing. We know that this has been a helpful source of information for decision makers who have not met Rob personally.

At the Rouge Valley Butterfly Garden, Tiffany and those around **her met together and contemplated possible routes of action.** In the end, she decided to **politely refuse** the garden label that had been offered, but make no other comment about the new gardener at the Centre. We felt that a decision had already been taken about the new garden and protesting it now might be hurtful to the new person, as well as unproductive. We decided that Tiffany's long track record of dependable and hard work would continue to set her apart in positive ways from other volunteers. She would meet and exceed expectations set for the other gardener. Furthermore, we would look for ways to broaden and deepen her participation and roles with the Rouge Valley so that she would eventually become even more than just the Butterfly Gardener. This all happened. Over the summer, it became clear that Tiffany's garden was thriving because she was there often and loved to be there. The new gardener seemed to have difficulty showing up and her gardening efforts were abandoned before the end of the summer. Tiffany eventually has taken on more and varied duties and deepened her role all around with the Rouge Valley organization.

As for the Day Camp, Tiffany's eloquent and sensitive Supporter had a **brief conversation** with one of the summer staff about how such segregated events just did not fit in with how Tiffany wished to live her life. Tiffany chose to volunteer as a gardener to demonstrate her love for nature, and she might choose any time of the week to be close to nature. Joining a group simply based on disability held no interest for her. This was a short and gentle conversation but gave the staff some things to think about. We simply **avoided** the Centre on Thursdays, no one reiterated the invitation, and the Day Camp folded at the end of the summer never to reappear.

The events of the Rougemount board not formalizing the Deohaeko seats is an example of a safeguard that might have been put in place but was not. In the end, we lost the opportunity to make the change and lost our seats on the board. We have come up with some new ways of remaining important within the community, and believe that **time and patience** will reward us with another opportunity.

Finally, in the story of the Supporter-sponsored segregated event, the strategy used was simply **if you have the power to end it, do so.** Given that the families have the ultimate say in how Supporters use their time, the message went out to all Supporters that such social events went against the thinking and philosophy of our family group and would not continue. A couple of people pulled out immediately. A couple of others went ahead, but with greater understanding. Then, in many one-to-one conversations with Supporters families clarified our values and the expected actions of Supporters. We told people that getting together with other folks with disabilities was an easy thing to do. Our family members have many opportunities to do so all of the time. What is harder and takes more attention, skill and dedication is figuring how to link the people they support to other people in the community. However, this work is also more vital to make sure people lead safe and secure lives. We reminded people that our resources for support were very limited and we preferred they turned their attention to the work that was harder, more demanding, and much more important.

The above stories outline many kinds of action.

Building Allies

A lifetime of valuing and building relationships and allies contributes to all of the above steps. "No man is an island entire to itself", stated John Donne. Just as we have to keep connections and relationships foremost in our minds for and with our sons and daughters, so we must do so for our family groups, small organizations or like-minded others with whom we feel strong. These allies will help us to be aware of what we have, keep vigil over future threats, and provide us with information, resources and strategies at times of crisis.

Looking back now, I can see that many of the strategies and approaches that fall into these four kinds of action that keep us safe, were in play in Durham Region that cold winter. The shock of the actions of the board of directors of the local agency was that many of us could not believe it had actually happened. At the time, and certainly within the first week, I would have said that we had safeguarded little and no strategy was in place. At a later point, however, I could see the situation in a different light.

For the past many years (ten or more) there have been at least two strong organizations that support the kind of thinking that we do. This has been vital in a number of ways. Whenever like-minded individual families or situations would come to the allocations table, or other places for funding or resource requests, there was a good chance that at least one of these organizations had a regular place at the table. They truly understood the work that we were trying to do and helped us describe our goals and dreams to other less sympathetic voices at the table.

Also, these two organizations working in partnership in the community were able to successfully submit many funding proposal to government, provincial association, Trillium and other funders in order to undertake projects which further supported the work that we did. Such projects might introduce like-minded families to each other for mutual support, or pilot innovative ways of people connecting and being a part of their community. If we did not always benefit directly from these projects, we did so indirectly by proceeding with our goals and work in a community which fostered and became aware of many similar endeavours. Many community members came to see connecting and volunteering and working in the community as just the way things were meant to be for citizens.

Additionally, within their own resources or those that they were readily able to attract, one or both of these organizations was able to provide a series of related (in spirit at least) training and learning events in the community. This gave rise to families, paid Supporters and staff, community members and others coming to speak in a common language. It also increased the ability of the whole community to see itself as capable and strong enough to include all of its members.

This is what we had enjoyed as a community/political climate for some years prior to this incident. It wasn't perfect, to be sure. There were still many other community groups and community organizations who continued to peddle a more segregationist-type of agenda—separate schools, separate places of work, separate housing for those seen as different or disabled. But those of us who thought in a different way and who were doing things differently in our small and quiet ways had two large, vocal and effective organizations who lent legitimacy to our way of viewing community.

So, I think that there was a good level of awareness of what this organization under its particular leader meant for many of us. Many people were vigilant, and there had been much talk among the allies of the possibility of this and subsequent actions taking place. Yes, we were powerless to stop it. But we were also remarkably prepared with several levels of response. An immediate team set up quick and effective phone trees to get the word out to families, members, and many supportive allies in many other organizations. One large, vocal group took to making a formal and orchestrated protest of community members (with a special out reach to families) to the board of directors and the Ministry. This was not in the hopes of changing their mind, but to register our protest that this was not an action that represented many members of that agency membership. One group figured out ways of protecting a couple of very fragile individual situations that were felt to be at risk. One group figured out ways to protect a series of commitments to value-based training events over the next three months. When that strategy failed, another couple of people figured out another way. Busy people came together at all hours of the day and night and figured out the important steps. Over time, small new groups have come together to protect or re-organize parts of the work that seemed most important to them. One group of families came together to make sure their funding would be portable, and therefore left them free to have their dollars funnelled through a different organization. Another group of people began to become involved with province-wide training initiatives.

Safeguarding does not mean that the threat or action will not come to pass with much of the devastation predicted. It does mean that we can be prepared, have alternate plans and already envision a future day where the change will not threaten us in the same way again.

For several years, we were still in the reacting and re-building phase of this recent action, and even now, there is much work left to do as a result of that time. There was a long period of great risks and hardships for many individuals—people with disabilities who are being supported in unique and unorthodox ways, families who need to be helped to explore positive options, staff who have made hard decisions to leave, to stay, to resist. There were also the deep regrets of those who were left behind— those in agency services because they have no family and no voice to speak differently, and those families in the future who come to the door and are offered services instead of hopes and dreams, or waiting lists instead of lessons in being charge of one's own destiny. It was also very difficult to fit in all of this extra meeting and planning and communication at a time when we all were managing our own busy personal, family and community commitments and crises. But at the same time, there is hope remained strong.

That hope continues today, and we can see there was good reason to hope. There is hope and energy in doing the right thing, with friends and allies. There is hope and commitment in standing up to define community as a place for all. There is hope and creativity in finding new ways to do old things. There is hope and faith in new alliances in formerly unnoticed quarters. There is hope in renewed commitment to what we value and believe in. And we have gained in awareness, gained in new skills and resources for future threats, and gained in stronger relationships with our sisters and brothers in struggle.

Many of us within Deohaeko were involved in this situation and we brought much to Deohaeko from our recent experiences. We realize that we have already done some of the work that needs to be done. We have a good degree of awareness, we are fairly vigilant, we have some good resources and strategies, and we have never questioned our need to make alliances. The following is some of our thinking as a result of the threats that we see around us. It generally follows the four points made above. Our stories are our examples of what this term 'safeguarding' means to us.

We need to look around our environment and carefully assess what we value. What is invaluable and worth fighting for? For Deohaeko, this list would include a safe, secure and cherished home, a voice in the decisions in most aspects of what one does with their time, having life opportunities that mirror as much as possible those of gender and age peers in the rest of the community, friends, places of welcome and refuge in many typical community spaces (churches, associations, recreation, shops, homes, etc.), support and funding that allow people to enjoy all of the above.

If this is what we value, and currently are able to enjoy and experience many opportunities for this kind of life, we need to ask ourselves, what allows this to be so? What in the political climate allows this to happen? What features of our community provide for welcome and opportunity? This should happen at all levels of society both macroscopic (the big picture), and microscopic and personal.

Within a closer radius, what keeps people and their dreams safe and well includes many things. Rougemount Co-operative and its intentional community provide people with an opportunity to live in attractive, safe and affordable homes where they are in close proximity to typical members of the community. Danger threatens when co-operative members get too busy with their personal lives to take their board roles seriously or when the board becomes split and power becomes the dominant force, rather than consensus building.

One way of keeping the focus on community has been for Deohaeko families to intentionally select events happening at Rougemount and consciously turn them into full community events. We used our recent Christmas party as an occasion to invite many, many co-operative members which resulted in a full-swing community potluck. The key is that we do not just invite people. We ask them to come. We ask them to contribute. We ask their opinion on food. We call them when they do not arrive on time. And for some of them, we go to them and accompany them to the party. We make it happen and it is a great time and no one wants to miss it. There was great community spirit built that festive evening in the co-operative. We have done the same for a number of annual events over the past few years. It is intentional. It is neighbourly. It is fun, and it safeguards a bit of the intentional community spirit at Rougemount.

A recent move to download co-operatives from provincial to regional responsibility has provided us with many new concerns. Hard-won approval to house one person in two-bedroom units where circumstances warrant will have to be negotiated all over again. We have fought this battle before and we know the risks. We are more ready this time, and should we lose, we are well prepared with fallback positions that will protect the places that our sons and daughters call home.

Deohaeko Support Network as a board and a group of committed people to keep an eye on looking out for the big picture is another measure that keeps us safe. We all get embroiled in the details of our individual lives, which of course, do not only include this son or daughter with a disability, but other siblings and their life struggles, sometimes elderly parents, our own health concerns and more. When we come together as Deohaeko, it is the time to put all of the 'other' a bit to the side for the moment. It is a time to focus on the issues that affect our lives and communities through this one person—our son or daughter. It is very important for Deohaeko to always include a strong core of members that can step outside of themselves for this time and really think about what is happening in the world and what it means for us. We are now thinking of ways to increase our membership, or include new board members of choice in a mentor-style relationship—both for their future benefit, and in order to support our falling energies.

Following this, the very parents who started Deohaeko Support Network and spent hours and hours clarifying their values, writing their philosophy, designing written visions and life plans, and developing support circles are of great value to us as a whole. The safeguard is in the presence and ongoing work of these people. The threat is in the next generation to see whether parents have been successful or not in conveying the knowledge, the dedication, and the courage to continue on this path. We have more work to do to ensure that the vision is being passed on well to good-and-ready hearts. We have started to meet another six times per year in 'Gatherings' which are one-topic discussions designed to deepen our understanding of a given issue. And we have put in writing, the values, beliefs and principles which guide us and may do the same for those that follow.

Our version of individualized funding allows families and individuals to have great control over their day-to-day support arrangements while still allowing families to share with one another in times of need. Twice a year we ask each other who has surplus and who needs a bit more support funding The way in which we individualize our funding safeguards people's choice of paid Supporters, unique support arrangements, flexibility, and the ways families choose to orient and educate Supporters.. This has a great impact on how, when, where, and why support is offered. This is worth protecting and hanging on to.

Valued roles in valued community settings with welcoming, positive members of the community are one of the strongest ways of subtly sending messages to all of the community (other families, policy makers, politicians,) that people belong and are here to stay. At any time of turmoil, whether that is family troubles, lack of good Supporters, funding problems, etc., people's typical and valued roles are often threatened. Knowing that these are vital, and also knowing that the key threats to these roles are during these times of crisis, are perhaps two important steps to ensuring that these are safeguarded. Opportunities for people to work, recreate, join associations and clubs and contribute to community life need to have back up plans. We struggle hard and imperfectly in this area. When crisis hits support, a parent's health, or the rest of the family, we are not very good at hanging on to the roles people hold in the community. Despite its obvious impact Brenda has had a few periods of up to six months when she has had little or no presence at her community park site, for which she is the city-appointed environmental steward. Each time this stops, the damage is significant. Sometimes we manage it better for awhile. For example, when it became clear that Tiffany's baking business, *The Tiffany Touch*, could not operate as a viable part-time business at this time, her circle spent many meetings figuring out ways to operate at a lower level which still offered her some regular customers and orders and therefore a legitimate claim to the benefits that role had afforded her over the years.

Where circles are genuine and thriving, the individual is safer and able to dream more certainly. Circles that learn and grow to accommodate and accompany their core member will be a safeguard into an uncertain future. Personal, committed relationships which can and do grow out of circles (or despite circles) are the single greatest safeguard for your loved one. The threats to this safeguard are the many pressures that turn circle meetings into a duty to be performed, a technology or just another item in anyone's personal calendar. This takes particular vigilance and commitment on the part of at least a couple of circle members. Alive and vibrant circles can be messy, a bit out of control, and moving in many directions. They are also available to take on a crisis because of these same characteristics.

Ordinary community members who have become friends, colleagues, fellow participants and neighbours also provide safeguards to people individually. Even when these relationships appear to be new and not (yet) very deep, ordinary citizens often make a good effort to take care of one another. One family received a call from an acquaintance of their son that he was seen without support in the mall. Neighbours offer rides for emergency appointments. Colleagues in work situations help solve problems, call family when a ride is late, and keep an eye out for people they work with and have come to know. We have many examples of ordinary community members reaching out to offer a helping hand.

Finally, the connections that we as individuals and as a family group have built up and nurtured over the years provide our biggest safety net. These include other family groups, our many allies within Durham Association for Family Respite, Peter Dill, supportive workers of various kinds working independently and even within service agencies, the various participants of the Values group, a number of professionals that we can count on for training, consultation, advice and information at all times (too numerous to mention), the Trillium Foundation especially in the spirit of our program manager who understands what we are all about, the Community Foundation of Durham Region, unique Supporters who have redefined commitment and vocation, and those family members who follow us on our rocky path.

As long as we are able to build and sustain such nourishing relationships as these, we will be able to live and dream and meet most of the challenges of our current society.

Chapter 10
Dancing in the Garden of Life

This chapter is dedicated to Marje Mitchell,
(1931-2003)
parent, friend, board member, ally,
who allowed us our first test of strength
into a future without a parent.

We are dancing in the garden of life. This is the analogy that I use for understanding where we are right now and what may lay ahead.

We are right where we want to be. Not everything is perfect, but we are where we want and need to be in order to make sure that life happens well for all of the people that we care about. We are dancing away in many parts of the garden of life with passion and flair accompanied by partners that are the envy of all.

First of all, we are present. This is important, but in many ways, this is not particularly new. In our first book, *We Come Bearing Gifts*, we celebrated being present. Presence is important, however, and cannot be taken for granted. It must always be a focus of our attention.

It is not uncommon for many people with disabilities to be seen as weeds in the garden of life. In so many instances, these people are ripped out the garden and cast aside as not belonging. The more the weeds are cast aside and not appreciated for their own features, the less we are all able to see the unique beauty and gifts that they surely have to offer. And what is a weed, but a flower that one does not want or whose beauty one does not recognize? All of the individuals of Deohaeko have experienced their presence being denied, being pushed away as a mistake, or being referred to a segregated program that is thought to be more 'appropriate'. Our first few years together were a celebration of getting beyond 'weed' status and helping others to recognize the beauty and value of our gifts.

Then, we were present in ways that allowed us to observe and appreciate the beauty of the garden, without really being part of the garden itself. I call this kind of presence, being wallflowers that surround the outer edges of the garden, but not being a full part of the life of the garden. People like to point to wallflowers now and again, but it is generally accepted that their place is along the edges and efforts to move into the centre of the garden with new partners and in new combinations may be rebuffed. Wallflowers do not really belong to the garden itself.

We are now present in ways that go far beyond being the wallflowers of the garden, admiring the beauty and life within from its outer edges. We are now part of what makes the life and beauty of the garden. We are part of the wild and unpredictable tumult of a thriving garden of life. We have figured out what parts of the garden would most welcome our presence, how to be present in meaningful ways, how to make contributions that the garden can honour, and how to build relations with those we meet. We spring up in all kinds of places, and our presence is seen as natural, or even as making a contribution to the patch that we adorn.

I see that our fragility is protected by the rough and tumble elements of many stronger, more vigorous species in the garden. At times our very frailty is what calls others to our sides. At times, we find that the more nourishing soil to welcome our presence is alongside of the hardy, tested varieties that have a perennial place in the garden. In any event, the juxtaposition of fragile and tough lends a new dimension to the garden, one that is noticed and admired by many who pass it by.

We are dancing in the garden of life, though it too, is fraught with dangers. Life is like that. The greatest of joys and possibility grow within that garden, but so, too, do all of the dangers that lurk in the world of humans. There are dangers from within the garden itself. The purple loosestrife, the dog-strangling vine, and other invaders threaten the presence of fragile plants. They are like those who do not extend welcome, or seek to push us to specific patches of the community where we are supposed to grow. They are those who would seek to relegate us to wallflower status if they could, or to choke us out all together.

There are also the dangers from without—pollution, unplanned urban growth, detachment of humans from the nature of life. These are a threat to the whole garden, but often they pose an even greater threat to fragile, vulnerable species first. In this way, our fragility is the gift that we bestow upon our garden of life. Like an advance warning of dangers ahead, evidence of struggle of the fragile ones in the garden can warn the whole community of dangers to their own health and survival. Our presence ensures that plans are made that protect and enhance the whole garden of life. We are all stronger when the most vulnerable among us are thriving well.

Despite the dangers there is hope. Each Spring finds the garden of life growing and thriving, working together to push forth and finding new ways around the threats to our ability to create together. And we know that, struggle as we might for our place and our survival in the garden of life, there is much greater hope for us here than ever there was as a wallflower on the outer edges where danger strikes first, or on the compost heap with those discarded as weeds.

As in many dances, we do not have all the partners we would wish for in the garden of life. But we do have partners, and the variety and choice of partners is much greater today than at other times in our lives. Many of our partners are strong, well-loved garden varieties that carry us forth into the dance in ways that display our talents and gifts in new ways for others to see. Gifts that may have been hidden when we stood alone, now shine against the backdrop of these partners.

Our most committed partners at the dance are past full bloom, and that gives us all cause for thought and reflection. Who will come to grow alongside and take their place? We think several new plants may have to grow where now only one is rooted. The wisdom and learning of the parent plant is not easily replaced. We wonder what we might need to do to nourish the soil for vigorous new growth. We wonder too, how to sow a common understanding of this vision of a full and lush garden, replete with all varieties, no matter how unique and rare their contributions. We will need to protect the integrity of this original seed stock.

The answer may lie in the soil which carries next year's seeds and protects dormant roots. In Winter, the garden of life lies still, preparing for the coming Spring. The roots wrap around each other and form common barriers against the frost and blight. Deep in the soil, deep within the roots, lies the memory of the garden that could be. It's the roots that need protection most of all. The roots carry the full story. They remember the ingredients necessary in the soil, the vital importance of belonging, the tools and strategies to create the garden, and the secrets to over wintering well. When the roots are well cared-for the garden will come to life again.

And we'll be there, dancing.

Three Phases to the Future

I look back over the twelve years (at the time of this writing) since Deohaeko Support Network first began, the twelve years since receiving charitable status, the eleven years since the first bit of funding, and the ten years since first moving into the newly built Rougemount Co-operative. I often think about life and the work happening in three kinds of phases.

The first phase was all about arriving. That was the building of the group, the designing of what 'home' might mean initially for people, the moving into people's co-operative homes, and the building of how people would live their lives. In the middle of our arriving, was the belief that the individual person came first. Arriving at the doorstep of life was defined in terms of that person and their hopes and dreams as near as we could discover them. We believed that our community would be better and stronger when all of its members, these individuals among them, were included and involved. We learned some very valuable lessons in those years that continue to help and guide us to this day.

The next phase, which is the central focus of this book, is all about exploring and deciding within this new life, ways that will help people establish deep, enduring roots while living a full, active and meaningful life as part of their community. We had to figure out how to get things done and keep things moving in positive directions. We began to realize that we need to make sure that life happens well in the middle of crises. We cannot afford to wait for critical times to pass before going on with people's lives. Crisis defines much of people's lives and we have to learn to work with these times as opportunities to learn. We began to understand that our greatest strengths are the allies and relationships we all form, the positive roles that we help people to enter into, the building of strong, knowledgeable support that keep things moving well. We saw for ourselves the strength of planning for and with people based on their interests and potential contributions. We began to see our communities as more open, tolerant and welcoming.

And we are now entering into a third phase. This phase is all about sustaining the structures, the thinking, and the support that has made many good things possible for our family members. This next phase makes us think about securing the financial future for our family members. It reminds us about the vital importance of building the relationship future now that will ensure a good life for our family member. And finally, it is an awakening to the fact that we must do all of this at the same time as repeating everything we have learned in the first two phases again and again. We must continually remind ourselves and teach significant others the importance of our first two phases' lessons.

Most of this book is about events and stories that took place up until the middle of 2003, but at this point, we will explore two areas that have their roots in the beginning and middle phases of our story, but which will define the shape of the third phase and its journey in significant ways. We have long felt that our future would be most positive if we were to find ways to both secure the financial future for our family members with disabilities, and to secure their personal lives through genuine, caring, committed relationship. Our efforts in these two areas are worth discussion.

Securing the Financial Future

Funding from government sources has not changed much in the past ten years. Our annualized funding which became firm in 1996 has remained more or less constant except for portions given up as individual families have left Deohaeko. On two occasions we have received a few extra dollars (amounting to a few hours per month for one or two individuals each time) when a local agency was in a position to do so.

Our Ministry dollars continue to be directed to Deohaeko Support Network through the Durham Association for Family Respite (a local transfer payment agency) and we re-direct monthly payments to each family as pro-rated in our original individual support plans (first written in 1996). We often call this 'fake' individualized funding because we individualize it, even though the government does not. We also continue with our practice of sharing the money among the families of Deohaeko as support needs change during the year. Families regularly talk to each other about who might need a few more dollars and who might have a few extra dollars to give. These are then given to each other from their own monthly allotment. In April of each year, each family returns to its constant original allotment.

Each family manages its own support dollars for themselves. They use the money to hire Supporters and direct their time as they see fit, according to our understanding of what a person requires and the goals and dreams of the individual. Families are required to keep records of this money and do so in a variety of ways. Most families handle this directly, some using a co-signed bank account with their son or daughter. In one situation, a daughter-in-law is now managing the money. In another, a second family has taken over the minimal record-keeping that is required. In a third situation, a mother has set up a system managed by the Supporters themselves, with enough checks and balances to ensure accountability. We represent enough different experiences and abilities with money to explode the myth that families cannot manage the paperwork that accompanies individualized funding. For us, it is a matter of principle. When families hand out the cheque, they are in charge.

There have been no extra dollars for rate increases or benefits over the years. Nonetheless, we decided on an increase in basic Supporter rates in early 2000, with an additional tiny increase after two years in appreciation of long term Supporters. This has added a $20,000 deficit to our budget every year. We use fund-raised dollars to cover this deficit.

We have been fortunate with our dollars and funding in several ways. In the first place, we built in an allotment to pay a family coordinator right from the very beginning. When we did not receive the initial dollars that we requested in the early years, we did not cut out the coordinator position, but rather carved a small piece from individual budgets to cover this position. This has grounded a coordinator position for our whole family group in our history and our funding. When we report quarterly to the transfer payment agency (and thus, the Ministry), we are careful to include the coordinator as a separate line item, in the belief that it is important to establish this within the core of our funding.

We have been able to secure small amounts of crisis or one-time funding for certain reasons, and this has occasionally boosted the amount of direct support available during a difficult time. Having a coordinator available to draft and coordinate the preparation of quick proposals at these times has been helpful.

We have been able to secure two Trillium project grants over the past eight years. One was a small project to help us think about individualized funding and to prepare a how-to manual, *Individualized Funding*, for ourselves and others. The second was a five-year project on sustainability. This project entitled, *Our Presence Has Roots*, has enabled us to research, establish and begin to fill an endowment fund for the future (see below). Our book, *On Our Own...Together*, records our research into many forms and possibilities of endowment, and our eventual decision. A second part of this project was to look at the ways in which people lived their lives and made connections and contributions while becoming a part of their community, and this book is the culmination of that part of the project. Although the Trillium projects do not provide us with direct support dollars, they have enabled us to be conscious of our learning, and have supported us to put this in writing for others.

In September 1999 we seized an opportunity to run a weekly Sunday morning Bingo. This enables us to meet our annual deficit and contribute a very small amount to long term planning. We are well aware that this is a short-term, energy-draining solution to a long term problem and continue to look for ways to let the government know that its funds do not currently meet our support requirements.

Our support requirements have not significantly changed from the first individual support plans that we put forth in 1996. However, we did not receive the full funding that we thought was necessary at that time. Like all families, however, we took the funding we could get and worked out ways for life to go on. This means that families have filled in the gaps in several creative ways. Families themselves have spent time with their son or daughter, in ways over and above what they would do naturally. This can mean spending a whole weekend day and night together, rather than a more natural evening visit, or figuring out several overnights among family members. Families have used a portion of their fund-raised Bingo dollars to add a few support hours. Families have accepted and welcomed opportunities from neighbours and roommates who have offered to spend time with the person for occasional or regular events.

We are clear that we have found ways to make the most out of inadequate funding over the years. We are even grateful for the opportunity that less than full funding allowed to leave space for natural supports to grow. This echoed a sentiment in our original support plans that no one's life should be supported by paid support 100% of the time.

At this point, however, we find that supports initially provided by the family (which is beyond the time that families always will spend with their family member naturally) are difficult to maintain at the same levels as earlier. Parents are ten years older than when we started out. Some are experiencing health problems, transportation problems, and they also need to share their time and energy with elderly relatives who also need their support. Donna has lost a mother, and gained a son. In the context of her place in her community, her support requirements have changed only a little, in terms of support dollars. Sisters and brothers, other family members and circle members are available to fill in some of the gap for each of the people, and do so now. However, most of these have young families of their own, and full or part time jobs that demand their time. Their time is more limited than that of parents, half of whom are retired or working part time. In some ways, more direct support dollars are required—our original support plans would be a great starting place.

For these reasons, we have developed a multi-layered approach to securing the financial future for our family members.

We are working hard with many families around Ontario to have the provincial government acknowledge and fund individualized support plans for people.

At the same time, all Deohaeko families have been engaged in a process of making out their wills and estate plans, in ways that will benefit their individual son or daughter. In most cases, Deohaeko will be given a clear role in supportive decision-making around their finances. For most people, this involves a Henson trust, and appointing people who know their son or daughter well to help with financial decision making (explained in detail in our book, *On Our Own...Together*. This does not address Deohaeko's deficit, but may secure individual's personal lifestyles and standards of living.

Finally, about five years ago, the families of Deohaeko Support Network, decided that ultimately the financial future of their family members would be most secure within our own hands. We set about securing a Trillium grant and have used it to research and establish an endowment fund with the *Community Foundation of Durham Region*. We are beginning to find ways to fill it, with our long term goal set at $5 million, or enough money to allow all support dollars to flow from the interest on that amount of capital. At that point, we will happily turn our current annualized dollars back to the government to re-direct it for other families who require the supports. We are currently very far from our endowment target and often our energies are taken away from this priority by the weekly Bingo, our own health and stamina issues, and the need to spend extra hours with our families members (beyond what we will always do naturally) due to support dollar shortages.

But we know that the dollars do not make sense without the context of relationship. In the end, what matters most to the individual will be the people who have chosen to be near to help make life's decisions and see them carried through.

Securing the Future Through Relationship

In March of 2003, our dear friend, fellow collaborator, and ally, Marjorie Mitchell died after a short intense illness in Ingersoll, Ontario. This has perhaps been the most serious event to us so far—a call to remind us of the importance of our path. For the first time, one of our children is left without parents. What does this mean for our group and the future of all?

We know full well what this means for us right now. We have spent countless hours over the years, not only sharing our dreams and our visions for a good future, but also our fears and our stating of the vulnerabilities. We know Donna well. Through Marje's eyes and Marje's heart we know her fragility, her vulnerability, and the very spirit of Donna that is worth fighting for. Only now it is passed over to us to fight and safeguard on Donna's behalf. Marje has allowed us our first test of strength into the future without a parent.

The task is daunting only because we want to do it so well. We want to do well for Marje. We want to do well for her daughter, Donna. We want to do well for her grandson, Matthew, and the promise of the next generation. But perhaps mostly we want to do well, so that in our turn this same will be done for our own.

This is our story for Marje.

Marje has a story to tell. But she is not here to tell it. She is gone since March 2003. She has entered that place that we must all go, but she's gone there before us. And in between her being here and one of us, and her going and leaving us, there is a story to tell.

It's the last family story—the one that no one wants to write. The one that says that I am now gone and others must go on. The one that says I've left behind what I've left behind—no more, no less.

For Marje, life was centred on her youngest two children, Donna and Bob, and her dear last-born grandson, Matthew. Her older son and family lived farther away, were well established and needed her less. That's the part of the story of her being here and one of us. We planned together, worked together, and solved countless problems together. We were creative, daring, and we aimed high. Life included supporting Donna to bring Matthew into this world and learning to mother him well. Life included figuring out with Bob what the next steps in his own life might be. Life included living in her own Rougemount apartment and living the life of the community. Life included being a part of the Deohaeko group in all of our early winter retreats, late night meetings, endless potluck dinners (Marje always brought the coleslaw), and glasses of wine in celebration of something very small. Life was centred in Pickering.

Sickness and death, however, took her away from us and to her older son, whom we did not know well, in Ingersoll, several hours away. Her going and leaving us showed us many painful gaps in our common understandings of what life would be like without her there. We knew Marje, but we did not know all of the family. She knew us well and trusted us in many ways, but important others in her family had not yet come to know us at all. There was no time to build that trust in the time that Marje had left.

How much time do we need to build trust among new family members? Four months in the middle of grief and loss was not enough. Twenty-three trips with Donna and Bob to Ingersoll, two hours away, always with another Deohaeko family member, coordinator, or friend to offer a ride and support was not enough. Months of sorting through stuff and wills, when we were wanting conversation, was not enough.

We heard Marje's wishes expressed over months and years of listening, choosing and talking it over with Donna. We shared the vision for a good life for Donna and Matthew that Marje had articulated over time. We understood her thoughts and hopes and dreams for Donna. We knew her fears, her concerns and her worries. We held it all carefully and carried it well. But we did not have a way to connect to family members outside of Pickering.

Today, a year later, our memories remain bittersweet. Our accomplishments are great. Donna has a good, committed circle which deals practically, if not perfectly, with the challenges and troubles as they arise. Matthew has started nursery school. Donna does a little bit of part-time work for the first time in three years. Donna and neighbours and friends find time every now and then to remember Marje in good ways. There is often a prayer for her and for Donna at the Rosary group. There was a tea on Marje's birthday, using her own porcelain tea cups. At another party, the last bottles of Marje's famous fruit liqueur were found and put out for friends who knew and loved her potion. At Thanksgiving, Christmas, and other holidays there are people to make sure that Donna has a place to be, or is helped to begin a tradition of her own. Donna has maintained and nurtured good contact with her aunt and uncle in Midland, and re-connected with an aunt in Brampton.

But family contact between members of Deohaeko families and Donna's family is more limited than it could be. Relationships between Donna, Bob and their family in Ingersoll are low key, and family there have little idea of the struggles and joys of life at Rougemount. There is perhaps much frustration and confusion on their side about a group who claim to know their mother so well. However, there is no coming together for learning or for planning. There are no conversations about what we can rely for upon each other. There is no common understanding of who we are and what we are all about. The opportunity for Marje to pass that along and form a real connection between the families of Deohaeko and this little known family member has gone. They are a part of Donna's family, but only a very small part of her life.

So Marje has left us with some gifts wrapped in a rough package of day-to-day messiness and problems.

The core gift, of course, is Donna. Donna knows more about relationships and how to grow them, and how to surround oneself with them than most people.

The next gift is that of not taking family for granted. We cannot assume that because we know the mother, that we know the children. We have spent so many long hours together deepening our beliefs, discovering new ways of thinking and discarding old forms that did not work. But we do not in return spend anywhere near the same number of hours talking to the children, the relatives, or even the circle members sharing our new ideas and helping them discover these new ways as well. We prepare ourselves well for the future but Marje reminds us that parents will not be there. If we understand the important things well and do not pass them along thoughtfully and carefully, others will have to start over again from scratch. The problem is that the parent is often the one that has the most status, the greatest possibility of reaching a sibling or a relative that has no connection with the rest of the family group.

The families of Deohaeko know each other's lives intimately and have pledged to help each other work out the future for their loved ones along the guiding principles upon which we have come to rely.

The final gift is still unfolding. Based on our experiences with Marje and her family, the families of Deohaeko have come together and outlined a process to help us move ahead based on what we have been learning. Our intention is to begin a series of conversations with the people who will carry on into the future. We want to begin the work of building a common vision of the future, based on the visions that parents with their sons and daughters have designed over the past years. We are not making any assumptions that family visions have been shared or understood with the members of one's family or circle. We know that this can not be taken for granted, and we need to begin at the beginning. We cannot yet report on the results of our intentions.

Some readers may read of the uncertainty of our path through the next phase and feel despair. They may wonder what good is all the work and the planning if at this late stage there is still such unknown. They see the hard work and the immense creativity that needed to be put into the first years in order to build a firm foundation, a soil that would yield results. They now understand much better all of the work, the planning and the thinking that has taken us through to this middle phase in order to help firmly establish people as growing, contributing and deeply rooted citizens. And here we are in all our success, achievements, and unfinished business, to announce that the lives of the people we care for profoundly are still incredibly fragile, and that their futures are not yet secure. The people—the single most important element to a positive and secure future—are just beginning to emerge and commitments are still untested. Some readers will gather these facts to themselves and will wonder if it is a worthwhile endeavour, a good place to put their time, energy and their love for their family member. In the end, people are still very vulnerable and we may lose it all.

To these readers I would share a few thoughts that motivate and give me energy. First of all, I think what the alternatives would have been had we not put our hearts, minds and energies in these directions. The sons and daughters of the families of Deohaeko have lived positive, hopeful, contributing lives for over fifteen years now because of this endeavour. The love, caring and joy that they had generated within their families for their early years has been shared with their greater community. Through our endeavours, they have been present to their families, their friends, their neighbours and their community in deep, meaningful and life-changing ways. They have taught us much, reminded us of much that we already knew, and built hope and new dreams within us all.

The alternatives to the kinds of lives they are now living would be a great injustice. The alternatives would not provide them with nearly the same degree of presence, voice, and ability to share their gifts.

Secondly, I think that regardless of the outcome of the journey, the path itself that we have chosen has been filled with love, joy, important lessons and vital opportunities that have given us strength and hope in many other parts of our lives. After all, we don't refrain from planting a garden just because we know that in the end winter comes anyway. We plant, cultivate, weed, and enjoy the garden in all of its stages.

Thirdly, I believe that each day that we are able to continue with our learning, growing, planning and dreaming is a day that we can tuck under our belts as an accomplishment.

Each day is a day that we would not have had to live and enjoy our lives in these ways that feel more right than wrong, that feel more about belonging than about being isolated, that allow people to be more often fully engaged and welcomed than wasting time. If things were to change drastically in some distant future, these days cannot be taken away.

Fourthly, I think that we have accomplished much that cannot be easily shattered. Individuals all know important things about their lives, their gifts and their dreams. They have the experience of having a voice. Enough significant others share this understanding that it will not be easily lost. Our foundations are sound and carefully built. Others will be able to follow the direction we have set, even if not our exact path. Other family groups will have learned and grown from our example so that our group in the future may also receive support from theirs.

Finally, I have come to know to never underestimate the richness of potential within community. It is often hard work to move against the tide of our human society. We need to observe that which is fleeting, discover that which is half-hidden, imagine that which is not yet possible, link with the few believers who are not easily identified, and dream that which is not yet desired by the rest of human society. There are low points, lots of hard work, and many times when things just don't work out. The fact is, such is life for everyone.

Out of community and away in separate and isolated places, I can only guess that the low points are lower, there is little point to hard work, and there is no one to help. All of which means that vulnerable people are even more at risk and never return to be welcomed into the hearts of their former communities.

At the same time, within community there are incredibly beautiful happenings, so complex and intricate that we could never design or create them ourselves. These are happenings that are like gems of hope and joy that appear at unlikely moments, but often with timing that takes my breath away. These are moments in community— the hidden gifts that may appear at any time—but you have to be a part of community in order to receive them.

This past year presented one of these happenings as Donna struggled through the first year without her mother to guide, support and love her. She was missing her mother and feeling rudderless in her life. She tried in many ways with much support from her friends and circle to recreate the family she so missed. She tried to keep in touch with her brother and family in Ingersoll, but visits were hard for them to manage with their large family and its own obligations, and telephone contact only filled in part what Donna was missing. She worked hard at a good relationship with Bob who also lives at Rougemount, but as a bachelor on his own, he was in more need for family moments and less able to create them than she.

People in Donna's circle and life worked hard to hold Donna well, creating a place where she could struggle and grieve and feel moments of family and togetherness as she pulled the pieces of her life together. There was always a place for holiday celebrations at someone's table for Donna, Matthew and often Bob as well. Transportation was always worked out for them. At times, we helped her to use her home as the focal point of the family celebration and others came to her for the occasion. We helped her to begin small Christmas and Easter traditions for Matthew. We made times of remembering Marje in all of our times together. We helped Donna figure out ways for Matthew to remember Grandma by tossing flowers into her beloved Rouge River at the anniversary of her death. These thoughtful events helped to ease her pain, and begin to imagine life without Mom.

And then, just over a year after her mother's death, Donna's biological family found Donna. Two brothers, who look exactly like Donna, only learned of her existence a month before and they scoured the Internet and did their own bit of sleuthing to find her. Donna's life has been touched and altered by these two young men and their wives and children who live in nearby Oshawa. She has met her birth mother, her grandmother, a cousin, an uncle, and three step-brothers. There are others still to meet. Donna has been invited to family events, with promises for holiday gatherings that include Bob as well. We don't know the future of any of these new relationships, but the possibilities and the hope are endless.

The timing of these events leaves us breathless, and we are stunned by the love and care and potential for family that has re-entered Donna's life. We could not have planned this so well. This is a happening from the heart of a living, imperfect human community.

In the aftermath of the initial high emotions, a few things become clearer to me. One is that this would have happened so much differently if Marje had not joined with the families of Deohaeko so many years ago. Those years have given Donna so much confidence, voice and skill that she was well able to respond to, embrace and return the delight and hope demonstrated by her brothers upon their first meeting. In these years, she became the woman, the sister, they see today. She is a mother of a fine, active young son. She had learned to read and obtained a college diploma, which led to a working life for some years. She had acquired a piano and is a pianist. She is a founding member of a large housing co-operative where she is loved and known and depended upon by many of her neighbours. She is a good friend to a wide circle of people who love her dearly.

Another thing that I learn from this event is that much of life is truly out of our control. The big events, the grand changes, the life-altering moments I can do little about. But there is still a very significant role for each of us to play. We can make the right decisions with the right people for the right reasons most of the time. And when we live well for that which is before us, we are holding a solid foundation and providing a good place for people so that when the wonderful, unexpected and brilliant moments of life happen for the people within our circle, they are as ready and able as possible.

I think back to the decisions and plans that Donna's circle helped to make over the past three years. Each decision was carefully considered and made with a view to the best possible life for Donna and Matthew. Many times the plans chosen were not the easy ones, but ones that would take more work but offer a better alternative for Donna. We chose to support Donna's decision to have and bring up a child. We chose to take joint responsibility for the life and health of the baby rather than allowing Children's Aid a monitoring role. We chose to help be near her mother as much as possible in her last three months, while honouring Donna's wish to remain in her Rougemount home most nights (day trips only to the hospital 2 hours away). There are many more such decisions made slowly and carefully, trying to gather with the right people for the right reasons most of the time.

In my mind, I see that this way of making decisions cautiously while acknowledging the bigger picture and the likely implications, is a caring, respectful way of embracing and being with the person. This is our way to accompany Donna and help her be as fully herself as possible, so that when the richness of life offers her a gem, she is able to seize it and use it to the fullest.

In this way, we hold close in our hearts—and share with each other daily—many small stories, images and moments that remind us that even if each of these were the only outcome of this journey, it would have been worth it—for the person, for ourselves, for our community. The paths that we have chosen have the potential for many of these moments, both small and grand.

What's Ahead?

These are the two key areas for us to work on at this stage—securing the group of individuals who will dedicate themselves to relationships that will safeguard a good life for and with each person, and securing the financial future for the sons and daughters of the Deohaeko families. At the same time, our daily struggles continue to challenge us.

Finding and keeping good Supporters is an important part of continuing to help people be truly involved in their communities. We need to figure out good ways of finding people, some new, value-based ways of educating people (in addition to the orientations provided by families) and recognizing their contributions. We need to work out ways of paying people well, and contributing to their pension and health plans so they can afford to keep working with our families.

We need to keep connecting with other families across Ontario in order to remain strong, gather new ideas, and support a strong family movement across the province. Our experience shows that there is a place for family-driven, person-directed supports in our communities. It is good for our family member, it is good for our families, and it is good for our whole community.

The rest of what lies ahead is still unknown. However, recently we have had an opportunity to think about what has been essential in bringing us where we are today. In a recent presentation to our provincial Ministry, we reminded ourselves of the most important elements of our story to date:

> For our sons and daughters, and for ourselves, Rougemount is not a residential option. It is home. It is where people are hosts in their own home, co-operative members with rights and responsibilities, and good

neighbours to one another. There is no support service within the building, and no office for Deoaheko Support Network. Supporters work directly with people in their homes, and the coordinator has access to a telephone in someone's second bedroom area.

If Rougemount is about where people have chosen to live, then **Deohaeko Support Network** is about how they live their lives. We are a group of families who come together to think about and plan for ways that our sons and daughters might live good, full, and contributing lives at the heart of their co-operative and larger community. We think about and plan for supporting our sons and daughters to create a secure and welcoming home, to enter into a range of relationships with many people to keep them safe, and to explore a range of typical and valued ways to contribute to their community as citizens. We do all of this with a range of family support, assistance from friends and neighbours, and some consistent paid support.

We are not a service model; not an agency. Board members are family members. Paid Supporters work for each family separately. Each person's life is very unique and is supported as an individual. Families help their sons and daughters hire their own Supporters, plan their own schedules, and remain in control of their lives.

Our story is not about the co-operative, although this is a very nice place to live. It is about the **capacity of families** to be creative and innovative, to have a vision and follow it through. It is about intentionally developing community no matter where one lives.

What we know best is that families need the resources and flexibility to create and innovate. In this way, people will end up with a wide range of places to live within their communities in as many different arrangements as there are people.

At this stage in our lives, we ask ourselves, what is essential to our story? What are the vital ingredients that make it work?

First of all, it is vital that we families who care for our sons and daughters deeply, have a chance to come together and dream **a vision** based on love, possibility and contribution. We need that vision so that we always know where we are going; so that we can always teach those in the future what we have learned to be true; and so that we can seize the opportunity when it presents itself.

Secondly, we hold a number of **principles** that guide our work and our efforts. Two key principles (although there are more…) are:

- A belief in our sons and daughters and the gifts they have to offer, and that community is stronger and better for all when our family members are included.
- A belief that people with disabilities are better off, and safer, in community than separated from community.

These two principles lead us to intentionally develop the capacity of communities in which we live.

A third important element to our story is that we are a **group of families working together**. We have spent countless hours together—talking, discussing, planning, and working. We have a clear understanding of the vulnerabilities of our children, of the growing threats posed by our society's changing values, and of the fact that we are a small number of people going against the stream. However, we have come to share a vision of what is possible today and in the future, and although that vision is not valued or shared by the greater society, we believe that it is a vision that is good and right, not only for our children but for our whole community. We know each other's children very, very well. We know the support plans for each individual and have had input into every one of them. We support each other, and we celebrate together.

Individually, we would not be able to accomplish so much. Together we are better, stronger, and more creative.

A fourth key element of our story is **individualized funding**. We had funds that we could individualize. We simply took the chunk of funding given to us and allocated it across all support plans. The total amount was inadequate—a little more than half of our total plans. Due to our high energy and commitment as parents, our faith and ability to encourage natural support through friendships with others, and our unique sharing of dollars we have nonetheless been able to support our sons and daughters and to help them follow many of their life goals. With individualized funding, we can set our own priorities, innovate, share amongst ourselves and stretch as we see fit.

Our experience shows us that individualized funding means individual support plans, individual goals and dreams, individual homes, and individual lives.

A fifth essential element to our story is our commitment to finding funding for a **part-time coordinator** or facilitator. Our coordinator helps each family individually, and the group collectively, map out and hold a vision for the longer term, while making sure that what happens now is sound and thriving. For us, one part-time coordinator for our seven families is extremely important to helping us build circles of support, establish connections in the community for our sons and daughters, find and orient new Supporters, and plan a solid foundation for the future. That we have had the same coordinator for over ten years gives us the added benefit of shared history and vision.

Our experience tells us that a facilitator or coordinator must be hired by and work for the family or family group— that is, unencumbered by either agency or government association. This independent nature of the coordinator will ensure that the family remains in control of the priorities, goals, and life directions together with their family member.

This role is also instrumental in enabling our families to deal immediately and effectively with times of transition and change.

Full and thorough **support plans** for each individual are a sixth important element to our story. Although each plan is detailed and flexible, we maintain some strong beliefs. No individual is planned to receive paid support 100% of the time. Family and friends will always make up an important piece of the plan. Each support plan is very individual and distinct. There is no congregated or group support, and no sharing of paid Supporters between families.

Seventh, we focus on **presence and relationship** as two key ways of planning with and supporting individuals. People must first be PRESENT in their community in typical, familiar and valued ways—only then, will ordinary people in community come to know the person and welcome them as unique and contributing individuals. We know from our experience with the Rougemount Co-operative and in the Durham communities where people are active, that presence (as described above) will change community members' perception of the person with a disability and encourage them to welcome them as a true part of the community.

Once people are present, it becomes much more possible to help them enter into relationships with those around. Relationships with a wide variety of people who know them well and care for them deeply represent the greatest safety net, and ensure the best quality of life for our sons and daughters.

In the end, we know that we are on the right path when we look at the evidence of people's lives. Our sons and daughters are living full, contributing and meaningful lives within the heart of their co-operative and greater communities, and have done so for the past ten years. They hold a wide range of typical and familiar citizen, work and recreation roles. Several people own their own small business. They are connected to a variety of other people in casual and intimate ways. Many ordinary community members have been positively affected and touched by getting to know our sons and daughters. Their lives have been changed as well.

People living more interconnected, interdependent lives where tolerance, compassion and flexibility reign—this is the strongest evidence that our unique approach is working for our children and for our communities. As we see our sons and daughters growing and moving forward in their lives, we grow in our commitment and determination to *intentionally* build community where everyone is included.

I say that we are looking ahead with faith and hope. We know that people continue to be very vulnerable, and as our society continues on its path of consumerism, materialism, and blatant disregard for the value of all life, the people with disabilities that we love and care about will be ever more in danger. We know that the kinds of policies, rules and ideas that run rampant through tenuous funding dollars will erode the foundations that we have so carefully built up. We know that the future will be even harder than what we are working through right now.

But we must each individually and then, collectively, choose a path with heart. We know what is needed for the ways ahead. We know what we need to do right now— make the right decisions for the right reasons with the right people, despite the uncertainty. We need to acknowledge and safeguard what is good and right. We know that we have laid a good foundation. We know that we have helped and are helping people now to live good, full and rich lives. We know that their contributions to the life of community are important and significant even while they may not be fully understood by all people.

At the end of the day, we know that there are still many small moments to be grateful for. And we know that when life presents one of it rare gems of potential, we will be in a great position to take full advantage. At this stage this is where we are: Living life as fully as possible for the moment, poised to grasp opportunities as they come to view, as vulnerable as ever to the whims of the larger majority in the future, with imperfect relationships to safeguard and protect. It's not perfect, but it is often very good, it is very much alive and it is ours.

Postscript—In Gratitude

It is the myriad of small things that draw me so to the people of Deohaeko. In the small gestures, I am stopped in my tracks for the moment. In that moment, I am nourished, sustained and reminded of the truly important things in life. I become grateful. Being grateful comes like a prayer on my soul.

I am touched by the gentleness that accompanies small offerings. These are not the tides of great emotions or passions. These gestures are accompanied by gentle, gracious feelings of gratitude, simple pleasure, and quietude.

I have come to spend a short while with Rob. In the midst of a conversation with his companion while he is sitting by, our eyes meet and he smiles a beautiful smile. I return the smile, quietly, and wait a moment. Rob starts to laugh and we suddenly share a moment of surprising depth—a meeting of minds and souls.

These are often gifts given to me simply because the giver can. With support, experience and opportunity, people are able to choose, take action, and make decisions about many aspects of their lives. I am honoured when they choose me.

Donna calls me upstairs at the end of a busy day when I really need to be going home right away. I stop by in a hurry. She has baked cookies and wants to give me some for my family. Among all of the people she knows and loves, tonight she has chosen me.

Sometimes the gesture is a quiet window onto a small glimpse of the world that I might not otherwise see. Often these moments renew my faith in people.

I am at the restaurant where John spends a lot of time. It is hockey play off season and John is wearing several clothing items to support his favourite team, the Toronto

Maple Leafs. A group of rough and tumble outdoor workers in for coffee call him over to admire his scarf and hat. They offer him a seat and talk statistics and predictions with him for five minutes. From my seat, my faith and hope in typical members of our community is renewed and sustained.

Some small gestures are simply a request to focus on the moment, and the person and the gift of what is right before me—a reminder not to get lost in the future, when the present is all we ever have.

In the middle of future planning, scheduling, and problem-solving, Jon's sharp "Agh!" draws me back to him at this very moment. He reminds me that he has wishes and dreams right now, as well as for the future— one of those is to be noticed and important for himself at this moment.

In a busy world, intent on important pursuits and great feats, small gestures are a poignant reminder that small things touch us in real ways. These small moments sustain me and give me a warm glow inside in ways that the abstract steps necessary to affect larger change can never do.

I have been carrying my cotton bag with its broken strap for more than a week. "Fix it," says one. "Get a new one," says another. Then, as I turn to leave late one night from Brenda's, where I leave my bag in between meetings, she says, "It was me. I did it." She points to the strap now securely re-sewn in place. She has seen what the others see. But she, alone, has acted. This is the gift of Brenda.

These small gestures make me slow down and really see the person before me. I am often rushed with many things to do—phone calls to return, people to talk to, schedules to work out, planning to do. I need these gestures to return me to what really matters.

Tiffany looks at me intently and expresses a warm welcome that is uniquely meant for me. If I am rushed or uncaring about her at the moment, I will miss this moment. But I know her to greet her, to wait for her to digest and think about my presence, and then to provide a greeting that she designs uniquely for me in this moment.

Sometimes the gesture is simply saying, "I choose you" and I am overwhelmed by the rush of joy accompanying this gesture. This often happens when I feel too busy to take on another engagement or commitment, when my day timer is filled to bursting, and when I feel too much is being asked of me. But inevitably, "I choose you" is an invitation to a commitment that carries within it the sustenance I need. It always is linked to moments of direct human contact which inspire and revitalize me.

Caroline Ann invites me as her companion on her three-day retreat in another city. I am honoured. I am refreshed by the break. I am grateful.

Time and again, in the days that I spend among the people of Deohaeko, I receive small gestures offered in gentleness. I feel deep gratitude for:

...the gentleness of a shared laugh

...the warmth of gift made just for me

...a new and heart-warming window on the world

...the insistent demand to focus on the person

...a broken thing noticed and mended

...a made-to-measure personal welcome

...the honour of an invitation.

...this gift of gratitude.

Thank you.

Resources

Resources

Building Family Strategies. (2004). Workshop Series for Families in Durham Region—with accompanying binder of written material, sponsored by the Durham Family Network, Durham Association for Family Respite Services and Deohaeko Support Network..

Lifetime Circles – a new organization in Ontario that seeks to provide supports and resources to circles or support networks in order to keep them strong, healthy and working well.

Meaningful Day, What is a Home? and **Families for Social Value and Inclusion.** Workshops by Darcy Elks. A series of practical, value-based workshops for families and their allies.

Strangers in the House. Workshop developed by Jo Masserelli of the *SRV Implementation Project* in Massachusetts and Joe Osburn from the *Indiana Safeguards Initiative.*

Bibliography

Klees, Janet. (2002). *Friends for Life,* conference report from the 2002 retreat for families at Shadow Lake organized by Lifetime Circles.

Klees, Janet. (1996). *We Come Bearing Gifts: The Story of Deohaeko Support Network.* Scarborough, ON: PSD Consultants.

O'Brien, John. (1996). *Tell Me a Story of Deep Delight,* unpublished report for the Durham Association for Family Respite.

Race, David G. (2003). *Leadership and Change in Human Services: Selected Readings from Wolf Wolfensberger.* Routledge, New York.

Remen, Rachel Naomi, M.D. (2000) *My Ggrandfather's Blessings: Stories of Strength, Refuge and Belonging.* New York: Riverhead Books.

Schwartz, David B. (1999). *Who Cares?: Rediscovering Community.* New York: Random House.

Thivierge, Debra. (1999). *Individualized Funding: The Deohaeko Experience.* Limited edition publication. Pickering, ON: Deohaeko Support Network.

Van Bommel, Harry. (2002). *On Our Own...Together.* Scarborough, ON: Resources Supporting Family and Community Legacies.

Vanier, Jean. (1999). *Becoming Human.* Mahwah, NJ: Paulist Press.

Wolfensberger, Wolf. (1998) *A Brief Introduction to Social Role Valorization: A High-Order Concept for Addressing the plight of Societally Devalued People, and for Structuring Human Services.* (3rd edition). Syracuse, NY: Training Institute for Human Service Planning, Leadership and Change Agentry (Syracuse University).

Wolfensberger, Wolf. (2003) *The Future of Children With Significant Impairments: What Parents Fear and Want, and What They and Others May be Able to Do About It.* Syracuse, NY: Training Institute for Human Service Planning, Leadership Change Agentry (Syracuse University).

Uditsky, Bruce. "Natural Pathways to Friendship" in Angela Novak Amado's (1993). *Friendships and Community Connections between People With and Without Developmental Disabilities.* Baltimore, MD: Paul H. Brookes Publishing.

Index